An Introduction to Global He

T0074850

The field of global health is expanding rapidly. An increasing number of trainees are studying and working with marginalized populations, often within low- and middle-income countries. Such endeavours are beset by ethical dilemmas: mitigating power differentials, addressing cultural differences in how health and illness are viewed, and obtaining individual and community consent in research. This introductory textbook supports students to understand and work through key areas of concern, assisting them in moving towards a more critical view of global health practice.

Divided into two sections covering the theory and practice of global health ethics, the text begins by looking at definitions of global health and the field's historical context. It draws on anti-colonial perspectives and concepts, developing social justice and solidarity as key principles to guide students. The second part focuses on ethical challenges students may face in clinical experiences or research. Topics such as working with indigenous communities, the politics of global health governance, and the ethical challenges of advocacy are explored using a case study approach.

An Introduction to Global Health Ethics includes recommended resources and further readings, and is ideal for students from a range of disciplines – including public health, medicine, nursing, law and development studies – who are undertaking undergraduate and graduate courses in ethics or placements overseas.

Andrew D. Pinto is a family physician, and Public Health and Preventive Medicine specialist in the Department of Family and Community Medicine of St Michael's Hospital in Toronto. He is also a research fellow at the Centre for Research on Inner City Health in the Keenan Research Centre at the Li Ka Shing Knowledge Institute.

Ross E.G. Upshur is former Director of the University of Toronto Joint Centre for Bioethics, and a staff physician at Sunnybrook Health Sciences Centre. He is the Canada Research Chair in Primary Care Research and, at the University of Toronto, he is a Professor at the Department of Family and Community Medicine and Dalla Lana School of Public Health, Adjunct Scientist at the Institute of Clinical Evaluative Sciences, an affiliate of the Institute of the History and Philosophy of Science and Technology, and a member of the Centre for Environment.

To Kim, Olivia and Sara with great love for making all things possible.
– Ross Upshur

To my parents, Barbara and Brian, for the values you taught me,
and to my wife, Malika, for helping me to live them.
– Andrew Pinto

An Introduction to Global Health Ethics

Edited by

Andrew D. Pinto
Department of Family and Community Medicine, St. Michael's Hospital,
University of Toronto
Centre for Research on Inner City Health, Li Ka Shing Knowledge Institute,
St. Michael's Hospital

Ross E.G. Upshur
Department of Family and Community Medicine, Sunnybrook Health Sciences
Centre, University of Toronto
Dalla Lana School of Public Health, University of Toronto
Canada Research Chair in Primary Care Research

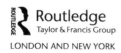

Routledge
Taylor & Francis Group

LONDON AND NEW YORK

First published 2013
by Routledge
2 Park Square, Milton Park, Abingdon, Oxon, OX14 4RN

Simultaneously published in the USA and Canada
by Routledge
711 Third Avenue, New York, NY 10017

Routledge is an imprint of the Taylor & Francis Group, an informa business

British Library Cataloguing in Publication Data
A catalogue record for this book is available from the British Library

Library of Congress Cataloging in Publication Data
An introduction to global health ethics / [edited by] Andrew D. Pinto and Ross E.G. Upshur.
p.; cm.
Includes bibliographical references.
I. Pinto, Andrew D. II. Upshur, Ross.
[DNLM: 1. World Health – ethics. 2. Healthcare Disparities – ethics. 3. International Cooperation. 4. Public Health – ethics. WA 530.1]
174.2 – dc23
2012022269

ISBN: 978-0-415-67352-5 (hbk)
ISBN: 978-0-415-68183-4 (pbk)
ISBN: 978-0-203-08222-5 (ebk)

Typeset in Sabon
by Saxon Graphics Ltd, Derby

Contents

Contributors

Kaosar Afsana
Health Programme, BRAC, Dhaka, Bangladesh
James P. Grant School of Public Health, BRAC University, Dhaka, Bangladesh

Kelly Anderson
Department of Family and Community Medicine, St. Michael's Hospital, University of Toronto, Toronto, Canada

Neil Arya
Office of Global Health, Schulich School of Medicine & Dentistry, University of Western Ontario, London, Canada
Environment and Resource Studies University of Waterloo, Waterloo, Canada
Department of Family Medicine, McMaster University, Hamilton, Canada

Abraham Aseffa
Armauer Hansen Research Institute, Addis Ababa, Ethiopia

Solomon Benatar
Bioethics Centre, Faculty of Health Sciences, University of Cape Town, Cape Town, South Africa
Joint Centre for Bioethics & Dalla Lana School of Public Health, University of Toronto, Toronto, Canada

Anne-Emanuelle Birn
Social and Behavioural Health Sciences and Global Health Divisions, Dalla Lana School of Public Health, University of Toronto, Toronto, Canada
Centre for Critical Development Studies, University of Toronto-Scarborough, Toronto, Canada

Adrienne K. Chan
Division of Infectious Diseases and Institute of Health Policy, Management & Evaluation, Department of Medicine, University of Toronto, Toronto, Canada
Dignitas International, Toronto, Canada
Global Health Division, Dalla Lana School of Public Health, University of Toronto, Toronto, Canada

Donald C. Cole
Global Health Division, Dalla Lana School of Public Health, University of Toronto, Toronto, Canada

Nathan Ford
Médecins Sans Frontières, Cape Town, South Africa
Centre for Infectious Disease Epidemiology and Research, University of Cape Town, Cape Town, South Africa

Lisa Forman
Global Health Division, Dalla Lana School of Public Health, University of Toronto, Toronto, Canada
Munk School of Global Affairs, University of Toronto, Toronto, Canada

Demissie Habte
Ethiopian Academy of Sciences, Addis Ababa, Ethiopia

Lori Hanson
Department of Community Health and Epidemiology, College of Medicine, University of Saskatchewan, Saskatoon, Canada

Jennifer Hatfield
Global Health & International Partnerships, Department of Community Health Sciences, O'Brien Centre for the Bachelor of Health Sciences, Faculty of Medicine, University of Calgary, Canada

Ghaiath Hussein
Department of Medical Ethics, Faculty of Medicine, King Fahad Medical City, Saudi Arabia

Athanase Kiromera
Department of Family and Community Medicine, University of Toronto, Toronto, Canada

Anant Kumar
Xavier Institute of Social Service, Ranchi, India

Maria de Lourdes Larrea
Universidad Andina Simon Bolivar, Quito, Ecuador

Victor A. López
Trauma and Global Health Program, Universidad de San Carlos de Guatemala, Guatemala City, Guatemala
Centro Integral del INCAP para la Prevención de las Enfermedades Crónicas, Guatemala City, Guatemala

Sarah Marsh
School of Nursing, University of Texas at Austin, Austin, United States of America

Jill Murphy
Faculty of Health Sciences, Simon Fraser University, Vancouver, Canada

Victor R. Neufeld
Canadian Coalition for Global Health Research, Ottawa, Canada

Stephanie Nixon
Department of Physical Therapy, Faculty of Medicine, University of Toronto, Toronto, Canada
Global Health Division, Dalla Lana School of Public Health, University of Toronto, Toronto, Canada
Director, International Centre for Disability and Rehabilitation, University of Toronto, Toronto, Canada

James Orbinski
Balsillie School of International Affairs, Wilfrid Laurier University, Waterloo, Canada

Jane Philpott
Department of Family and Community Medicine, University of Toronto, Toronto, Canada
Department of Family Medicine, Markham Stouffville Hospital, Markham, Canada

Andrew D. Pinto
Department of Family and Community Medicine, St. Michael's Hospital, Toronto, Canada
Centre for Research on Inner City Health, Keenan Research Centre, Li Ka Shing Knowledge Institute, St. Michael's Hospital, Toronto, Canada

Kevin Pottie
Centre for Global Health, Institute of Population Health and Bruyere Research Institute, Departments of Family Medicine and Epidemiology and Community Medicine, Faculty of Medicine, University of Ottawa, Ottawa, Canada

Katherine D. Rouleau
Global Health Program, Department of Family and Community Medicine, University of Toronto, Toronto, Canada
Department of Family and Community Medicine, St. Michael's Hospital, Toronto, Canada

Ana Sanchez
Department of Community Health Sciences, Faculty of Applied Health Sciences, Brock University, St Catharines, Canada

Malika Sharma
Department of Infectious Diseases, Division of Medicine, University of Toronto, Toronto, Canada

Jerome Amir Singh
Centre for the AIDS Programme of Research in South Africa, University of KwaZulu-Natal, Durban, South Africa
Dalla Lana School of Public Health, Joint Centre for Bioethics, and Sandra Rotman Centre, University of Toronto, Toronto, Canada

Janet K. Smylie
Centre for Research on Inner City Health, Keenan Research Centre, Li Ka Shing Knowledge Institute, St. Michael's Hospital, Toronto, Canada
Department of Family and Community Medicine, St. Michael's Hospital, Toronto, Canada
Dalla Lana School of Public Health, University of Toronto, Toronto, Canada

Ross E.G. Upshur
Department of Family and Community Medicine, Sunnybrook Health Sciences Centre, Toronto, Canada
Dalla Lana School of Public Health, University of Toronto, Toronto, Canada
Canada Research Chair in Primary Care Research

Foreword

James Orbinski

Global health in its broadest conceptualization connotes wellbeing in a state of justice. If global health is to be something other than an ideal perpetually beyond our grasp, it needs a framework rooted in fact, history, contemporary political reality and morality.

The primary factors that shape the health of citizens are not medical treatments or lifestyle changes, but rather the living conditions people experience and inequities in the societal determinants of health (Rasanathan and Krech 2011). A 2008 World Health Organization Commission concluded that 'social injustice is killing people on a grand scale' (WHO 2008: 6).

Addressing injustice and enhancing global health is a matter of practical action. It requires careful thinking, initiative and a willingness to experiment with new approaches. Most importantly, it requires that we think ethically and then act ethically. Ethics is not morality, but is dependent on it. Ethics demands that we are explicit about our moral frameworks and our choices, and that we explicitly explore the consequences that arise from these.

The purpose of ethical decision-making is not to provide a singularly correct answer or 'the Truth'. No one set of fixed rules will suffice to guide ethical choices, as most ethical issues cannot be pursued in a purely algorithmic way. There is often an inherent dilemma in weighing competing principles. Ethics allows us to initiate action with explicit moral reasoning and to evaluate outcomes from both objective and moral perspectives in order to improve our future choices and actions in the pursuit of global health.

This book is not about what perfect arrangements in global health may be. It is about how to think about and act toward achieving this ideal. It lays out power structures and traces their origin; it explores the dynamics of the challenges posed by global health; it identifies the moral goods that are at issue and how to approach their ethical consideration.

If the pursuit of global health is to avoid reinforcing and reproducing inequity and injustice – through, for example, the negative effects of good intentions – ethics must be central to reframing and reformulating our choices and actions. This book offers a masterful introduction to the ethical pursuit of global health and is a bold beginning to this necessary and good enterprise.

References

Rasanathan, K. and Krech, R. (2011) 'Action on social determinations of health is essential to tackle noncommunicable diseases', *Bulletin of the World Health Organization*, 89: 775–76. doi: 10.2471/BLT.11.094243

WHO (2008) *Closing the Gap in a Generation: Health Equity through Action on the Social Determinants of Health*. Final Report of the Commission on the Social Determinants of Health. Geneva: World Health Organization.

PART I
Theory

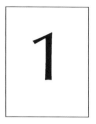

1 The context of global health ethics

Andrew D. Pinto, Anne-Emanuelle Birn and
Ross E.G. Upshur

Objectives

- To present a historical perspective on global health, using a political economy
  framework
- To discuss past and current definitions of global international health and relate this
  discussion to ethics
- To develop a rationale for global health ethics

A) Introduction

We live in a radically unequal world in terms of both health and its underlying
determinants. Even the most cursory review of the available data makes this evident.
On average, a person born in 2010 in Afghanistan, Chad or the Central African
Republic can expect to live to approximately 48 years, whereas the average life
expectancy is 80 years in the Republic of Korea, 82 in Iceland, and 83 in Japan (WHO
2011a). Globally, in 2009, approximately 8.1 million children died before their fifth
birthday, deaths occurring almost exclusively in low- and middle-income countries
(LMIC) (WHO 2011b). The vast majority of these are preventable deaths due to
diarrhea, pneumonia and malaria (Jones et al. 2003). It is estimated that in 2008,
358,000 women died in childbirth, with 99 per cent occurring in LMIC. This has
remained consistent 'year after year' and again, these deaths were/are almost entirely
preventable through existing knowledge, health services and interventions to improve
living conditions (Campbell et al. 2006).

Stark as these figures are, national averages hide within-country differences that are
even more striking. Evidence cited in the Final Report of the Commission on the Social
Determinants of Health (WHO 2008) demonstrates that the health of individuals and
communities is intricately tied to social factors. These include income, class, education
level, employment relations and race/ethnicity (Public Health Agency of Canada 2004).

To take just one determinant, in every country, the poor fare worse than the wealthy. In Scotland, there is a gap of over ten years in healthy life expectancy – years spent in good health – between residents of the most deprived and least deprived neighbourhoods (Wood et al. 2006). Similarly, the maternal mortality rate is three to four times higher among the poor compared with the rich in Indonesia (Graham et al. 2004), and in Peru infant mortality is almost five times higher in the poorest quintile of the population compared with the wealthiest (Gwatkin et al. 2007). Across the world, certain racial and ethnic groups fare worse than others living in the same country. In an oft-cited example, African-American men in Harlem, New York were found to be less likely to reach the age of 65 than the average man in Bangladesh (McCord and Freeman 1990). Indigenous peoples, referring to communities that share a historic link with pre-colonial societies, have lower life expectancies than their non-indigenous counterparts in every country where this has been studied (see Chapter 6). For example, Indigenous Australian men have a life expectancy at birth of 59 years, compared with 77 years for all Australian men (Australian Government 2009). In Canada, Aboriginal men live on average eight years less than the male population as a whole (Anderson et al. 2006). Such disparities between rich and poor nations, and between privileged elites and marginalized populations *within* each country, are expected to worsen with the negative effects of climate change (Costello et al. 2009) – which is likely to affect LMIC disproportionately – and by the fallout of the 2008 global financial crisis (Catalano et al. 2011; Stuckler et al. 2011).

None of these realities is new or surprising to health professionals, academics and policy-makers who are interested in global health. As never before, we have available an abundance of knowledge about such deplorable health inequities, a term referring to the differences in levels of health between groups in a society that are unjust, unfair and avoidable (Whitehead 1992; Starfield 2006). Further, tackling such health inequities has risen on the political agenda. In October 2011, representatives from 125 governments met at the World Conference on Social Determinants of Health in Rio de Janeiro, Brazil. The text of the conference's Political Declaration contains statements such as 'we need to do more to accelerate progress in addressing the unequal distribution of health resources as well as conditions damaging to health at all levels' (WHO 2011c: 2). Addressing social inequity is even entering the conversation at the 2012 World Economic Forum, where typically the focus is on economic growth and competitiveness (WEF 2012).

Given the evidence that significant, remediable differences in health exist globally, and that there is a stated goal to address them, what is being done? Clearly not enough: inequities in health have persisted – and even increased – despite enormous resources being channelled into reducing them, despite a rich body of evidence on effective measures, and despite strongly worded statements by international bodies that these efforts should be a top priority (WHO 2008).

This book aims to help you explore *why* this is the case and what can and *should be* done. Changing the systems that result in unnecessary death and suffering is a key goal of global health practitioners. Here we hope to move the reader from an intuitive sense that something is wrong to a deeper understanding of how power, access to resources, justice and fairness apply to health – questions with which global health ethicists are wrestling in an ongoing manner. This chapter begins by reflecting on what is meant by global health and how the field and its precursors have evolved over time: before solutions can be proposed to address inequities, it is essential to understand in what context they have arisen. Recognizing that there is a multitude of ways to address a problem, we then argue that ethical perspectives can contribute towards formulating responses – in terms of both avoiding doing harm and actually improving global health inequities. Finally, we highlight what the remaining chapters will cover as an entrée to engaging in global health ethics.

B) Historical roots of global health

'Global health' has entered into widespread use relatively recently and has been rapidly adopted, particularly in North America, as a field of study and practice. Yet whether it is even a new or separate field remains controversial (Farmer et al. 2009; Fried et al. 2010). Using the term 'global health' became common in the early 1990s, when the end of the Cold War appeared to open up new possibilities for health cooperation across countries to address problems of shared concern (Kickbusch 2002; Birn 2011; Bozorgmehr 2010). Among powerful players it has largely replaced 'international health', which in turn displaced 'tropical medicine' or 'colonial medicine' as the dominant term to capture the activities characterizing this field. Tracing the links between these conceptualizations is important to understanding the values and theories that underpin the field today.

Going back more than a millennium, outbreaks of plague periodically turned health into a regional or even a global problem, but until the rise of the modern state and a system of inter-state relationships, there was no organized mechanism to focus worldwide attention on health. By the nineteenth century, a confluence of developments – the most intense period of (European) conquest and imperialism, the industrial revolution, the concomitant revolutions in transport and global commerce, and the rise of modern medicine – forced sustained attention to health as more than a local matter.

Starting with Spain and Portugal's first invasions of Africa, South Asia and the Americas in the fifteenth century, the nations that established colonies in the so-called tropics were concerned with protecting soldiers, settlers and merchants from novel diseases that they were exposed to, both to secure their investments and to maintain their hold on power (Berlinguer 1992). As imperial enterprises became more permanent, colonial authorities also became concerned with maintaining the productivity of, for example, miners and plantation workers. Colonial powers set up medical offices and systems of regulation and intervention across their possessions to control epidemics, stave off uprisings, protect settler populations, and apply the disease-control tools of the day to 'civilise' subject populations (Birn et al. 2009).

Tropical medicine emerged in the nineteenth century, together with the new fields of bacteriology, parasitology and helminthology, closely related to the needs of colonialism (Arnold 1997). The development of this field was underpinned by the formulation in the colonial imagination of the 'tropics' as an exotic *other* (Said 1979) with purportedly distinct ecological characteristics. European and colonial tropical medicine institutes mounted field trials and measures focusing on epidemics and other health problems that threatened trade, productivity and the viability of colonies (De Cock et al. 1995). Religious missionary work and proselytizing was also closely related to the expansion of colonies and provided moral justification, especially through the building of hospitals and clinics and the provision of health services to indigenous communities as a key part of winning over the local population. For example, the Belgian regime in the Congo was extremely brutal, even as missionaries from a variety of countries helped it establish one of the most extensive networks of health clinics in any colonial territory. These efforts drew on European conceptualizations of indigenous peoples as weak, of different races being more or less suited for labor in the tropics, and of the racial superiority of people of European stock (MacLeod and Lewis 1998).

During the second half of the nineteenth century – at the height of the industrial revolution – the modern international health system was conceived, motivated by a growing (if divisive) belief that disease could spread rapidly through trade (e.g. the nineteenth century's repeated cholera pandemics) and the movement of people (in terms of large-scale immigration and the annual Hajj). Facilitated by a diplomatic context favouring state–state cooperation in the wake of the 1815 Congress of Vienna, most European countries recognized that the ongoing threat posed by epidemics to commerce and to their populations demanded some form of international agreement to reform quarantine measures (Harrison 2006). The first International Sanitary Conference was held in Paris in 1851, but inter-imperial rivalries resulted in little concrete action for several decades, even as the opening of the Suez Canal in 1869 shortened trade routes between Europe and East and South Asia (Bynum 1993). Finally, in 1907, the Paris-based Office International d'Hygiène Publique, mandated with the interchange of health information and the development and oversight of sanitary treaties, was founded. A fully fledged international health organization was founded after World War I – the League of Nations Health Organization (LNHO), based in Geneva. Drawing on social medicine approaches, the LNHO's ambitious agenda included not only infectious disease control, but also: vital and health statistics standardization and dissemination; running expert commissions charged with standardizing medications and vaccines; and studies of broad public health issues such as housing, medical education, health systems and services, economic depression, nutrition, human trafficking, rural hygiene, chronic disease, and the social causes of infant mortality (Borowy 2009).

By this time, an International Sanitary Bureau for the Americas had already been established in Washington, DC (in 1902, eventually becoming the Pan-American Health Organization in 1958), technically the world's first multilateral health organization. With the United States as the hemisphere's dominant power, and bolstered by its invasion and occupation of Cuba (justified largely as a means of controlling yellow fever), international sanitary agreement was easier to reach, especially given yellow fever's ongoing threat to commerce throughout the region. The renewal of the construction of the Panama Canal in 1904, key to the USA's global trade aspirations, further stimulated intra-continental disease-control efforts. Under French control since the 1880s, the project had stalled for decades after some 20,000 French and Jamaican workers died from yellow fever and malaria. A massive US military-led effort was marshalled to eliminate the breeding grounds of insect vectors, but it ignored the endemic problems of local populations such as tuberculosis and infant diarrhea. Once the Canal opened in 1914, there were renewed fears about – and redoubled efforts to control – the spread of communicable diseases through international trade.

A key player in this period was the Rockefeller Foundation, which helped popularize the term 'international health' through its influential International Health Board and Division (Cueto 1994). Launched in 1913, the Foundation pioneered cooperative public health efforts in almost 100 countries and colonies across the world through disease campaigns, support for public health institutionalization training, the establishment of schools of public health, and funding for thousands of fellows to pursue graduate study in North America (Birn 2006). This was the beginning of US-led international health 'philanthropy', foreshadowing and influencing the Milbank and Commonwealth Funds, the Kellogg and Ford Foundations, and the more recent Bill and Melinda Gates Foundation, which have substantially shaped the global health agenda. International humanitarian NGOs, such as the International Committee of the Red Cross (ICRC), established in 1863, also became active in this period. The ICRC was an important purveyor of care to refugees, wounded combatants and other war victims during World Wars I and II. It also played a significant role in shaping ideas about ethical standards during wartime, especially through the Geneva Conventions, although the ICRC has been critiqued for not having taken a stance against war itself (Hutchison 1996).

'International health' thus began to replace tropical medicine in the early twentieth century, related to the rise of internationalism and cooperation between nations. Like tropical medicine, international health emerged from a worldview where metropolitan centres – the imperial powers in Europe, North America and Japan – extended significant influence to their peripheral colonies and former colonies, patterns that were resisted in a variety of ways. Initiatives framed in international health terms often served the political and commercial interests of the dominant nations, but were also caught up in rivalries between major powers. Despite the optimism with which the United Nations (UN) was established in the wake of World War II – and the founding of the World Health Organization (WHO) in 1948, its sister UN agencies, and a range of bilateral and non-governmental organizations with a wide purview over international health (and development) activities – the international health arena became embroiled in the competition between the Cold War's superpowers. For almost half a century (1946–91), the US-led Western bloc and the Soviet-led Eastern bloc competed for allies and support among the 'non-aligned' countries of the Third World, with health frequently utilized as a foreign policy pawn in this effort (Packard 1997). Notwithstanding these pressures, in 1978 a broad coalition of public health actors across the world committed themselves to the goal of 'Health for All by the Year 2000' at the largest international health conference ever held, under the auspices of WHO and UNICEF in Alma-Ata in the former Soviet Union (Brown et al. 2006).

The end of the Cold War in the early 1990s was a mixed time for international health efforts. On one hand, a much hoped-for peace dividend gave greater prominence to influential humanitarian NGOs, particularly Médecins Sans Frontières (MSF, founded 1971), an organization that literally emphasized a borderless world (see

Chapter 11). However, the growing dominance of neoliberalism, the globalization of trade, and the influence of the World Bank and wealthy nations shaped international health priorities in a different direction. WHO lost (control of) much of its funding, and it was compelled to return to more traditional disease control efforts (Walt 1993), although the founding of UNAIDS did portend more ethical and collective approaches to addressing HIV/AIDS (see Chapters 4, 5 and 11). Further, after the attacks of September 11, 2001, health once again became part of the USA's and other Western nations' security agenda. The spread of disease in LMIC was now framed as a potential security threat to high-income countries (HIC) (Gow 2002).

C) Global health today

Global health is the current paradigm of health cooperation between nations and multilateral organizations, particular to contemporary political, economic and social arrangements, but also unavoidably retaining historical antecedents in tropical and colonial medicine and international health (Macfarlane et al. 2008). A single definition of global health remains elusive. For example, the US Institute of Medicine defined it in 1997 as 'health problems, issues, and concerns that transcend national boundaries, may be influenced by circumstances or experiences in other countries, and are best addressed by cooperative actions and solutions' (Institute of Medicine 1997: 11). This evolved into a 2009 definition of 'the goal of improving health for all people in all nations by promoting wellness and eliminating avoidable disease, disabilities, and deaths...improv[ing] health in low and middle-income countries' (Institute of Medicine 2009: 1). As Birn et al. (2009) have noted, there is a clear relationship between the popularization of 'global health' and the term 'globalization'. For example, academic health science centres in HIC often view global health as a way to operationalize 'global agendas' (MacLean and MacLean 2009; Crane 2011) (see Chapter 9). Globalization – the increasing interconnectedness between people, but also the powerful influence of global neoliberalism – has had a profound impact on the health of populations (Labonté et al. 2011). It has influenced which interventions have come to dominate global health, shaped by the role of market forces to address health needs (WHO 2012) and the emphasis on delivering technical solutions to improve population health (Larson et al. 2011).

An influential definition that has been taken up widely is:

> global health is an area for study, research, and practice that places a priority on improving health and achieving equity in health for all people worldwide. Global health emphasises transnational health issues, determinants, and solutions; involves many disciplines within and beyond the health sciences and promotes interdisciplinary collaboration; and is a synthesis of population based prevention with individual-level clinical care.
>
> (Koplan et al. 2009: 1995)

Other definitions, including 'the health of marginalized populations, wherever they exist' (Pinto and Upshur 2009), have tied global health to human rights more specifically (see Chapter 4) and speak more directly to upstream determinants of health. Many of these definitions are silent about the underlying causes of inequity, and do not speak to issues of power and resistance that are so essential to how change takes place (Birn 2011). The root causes of health inequities relate to the complex issue of how power and resources are distributed globally, and how this (unfair) distribution is maintained by a range of political and economic forces (WHO 2008). Definitions that ignore these matters are particularly unhelpful when considering the ethics of global health.

As such, global health is a contested term used mostly by academics, health practitioners and donors in HIC to describe activities that previously were labelled tropical medicine or international health (Benatar and Upshur 2011). Still, because the stated goals of global health typically include reducing health inequities and achieving health for all – reflecting roots in public health and the influence of the human rights agenda – and because it is now pervasive in North America, we use the term 'global health' in this book. Efforts that are labelled global health span a wide range of activities, from technical solutions at the molecular level to population-level interventions, and cut across a variety of academic disciplines and health professions. Just as was the case with tropical medicine and international health, such interventions and activities are heavily influenced by the social, political and economic philosophies of those who fund and direct them. This also means that they have the potential to incorporate ethical perspectives.

Global health today is a complex field of practice, involving thousands of individuals who come from an enormous number of disciplines conducting work with communities in both HIC and LMIC. Such activities occur through a myriad of actors with multiple and often conflicting motivations, including academic centres (typically in HIC, increasingly in partnership with institutions in LMIC; see Chapter 9), NGOs, government agencies and community service agencies. This work is supported by a large pool of funds (McCoy et al. 2009), reflecting the strategic interests of high-income governments (Ollila 2005), as well as trans-national corporations, philanthropic institutions and international financial institutions such as the International Monetary Fund and World Bank. Understanding the connections among academics, development workers, humanitarian NGOs, funders and governments can prove difficult, particularly when attempting to decipher who is responsible for what (see Chapter 5). Global health involves an overlapping and shifting mix of research, development work, humanitarian assistance, clinical work, business, public health, advocacy and political engagement (see Chapter 11). As an area of scholarship, global health is attracting more and more students who engage in research and practicum placements – called electives or international service learning – and who increasingly seek formal education to become global health practitioners (see Chapters 3 and 12).

D) Political economy of health

Global health academics, professionals and educators concern themselves with a multitude of interconnected problems. We propose a **political economy of health** model (Navarro 1981) to begin to categorize these in a way that makes sense. As Birn et al.

(2009: 134) note, this approach 'considers the political, social, cultural, and economic contexts in which disease and illness arise and examines the ways in which societal structures interact with the particular conditions or factors that lead to good or ill health'.

At the **individual level**, let us imagine a common clinical scenario: an infant in a LMIC is seen in a clinic run by a humanitarian NGO. She is diagnosed with pneumonia and requires an antibiotic. This medication is readily available in resource-rich settings but not where this child is living. This is seen as a problem – perhaps because it is considered unjust or unfair that this child should die for lack of a cheap, simple treatment – and the solution proposed is to deliver this antibiotic to the child when she needs it. Such a seemingly singular problem of access to care rapidly becomes several things to consider that continue to fall within the scope of global health. Were the way in which the child was examined, the diagnosis suggested, and the treatment recommended culturally appropriate? Do they 'translate' for the caregivers? What about the ongoing care of this child, such as dealing with an allergic reaction to the antibiotic? How will follow-up be ensured in case the medication does not work? What about a vaccine that could have prevented this bout of pneumonia? Is the infant predisposed to such infections because she is HIV+, and could this have been tested for, treated – or even better – averted through prevention of mother-to-child transmission programmes?

Thinking about the **family level**, did the caregivers/family have to pay a user fee to access the clinic? Did they have to travel a long way, take time off work and pay for transport? How does this infant's risk of pneumonia relate to whether or not she was breastfed? Or to the living conditions, income and education level of her mother? Does the income level of the father/household relate to the nutritional status of the child? What about the family's access to clean water and sanitation? Do they have other children who are ill, what is the size of the family, and is their home crowded? Does the gender of this infant influence the way her family influences her access to care and resources? Do all children in this family have the same access to education? Are there cultural or religious issues involved in these matters?

At the **community level**, is pneumonia common? What other diseases are prevalent, and why? What are the conditions of the neighbourhood and region in which this family lives? Is there access to schools and sources of employment? Why was there no access to government-supported health services locally? Is there a pharmacy nearby where the antibiotic could be obtained? What are the broader societal determinants of health (Birn 2009), including work conditions, transport services, conditions of sanitation, housing and overcrowding? What resources are available to pay local health providers to staff the clinic? Is this community seen as important in the eyes of the national government, or is it relatively neglected compared with other regions? Are there many global health organizations in the community, what do they do, and what has been the past experience with these or similar organizations? Will the presence of this NGO clinic create conflict with local traditional healers?

At the **national level**, what is included in the social policy agenda, and what measures exist to protect low-income populations? How are the most marginalized reached? Who owns and controls national resources? How does the government decide where to place health clinics and hospitals? How does it decide on salaries for health workers, and how is this constrained by the national budget? And by lenders such as the

International Monetary Fund, World Bank, regional development banks and commercial banks? What is the government policy around essential medicines? And how did the national government come to power? How is political power distributed (Navarro 1981)? Is there a system of accountability to voters? Is corruption prevalent? What are the class/race/gender structures of ownership and the labor force? Is health – and its determinants – seen as a human right, and, importantly, is there enforceable legislation to protect this right? Are there civil society organizations active in this area?

At the **international level**, is this country an ally of wealthy and powerful countries, including emerging middle-income countries? Can it influence trade policies? What does it produce and what does it buy and sell on the international market? How is it affected by the practices of certain HIC, such as the recruitment of health professionals? What is the impact of international treaties on the patenting of drugs, food subsidies, social rights, the movement of refugees and addressing climate change? What is the role of advocacy groups in creating change around some of these 'upstream' determinants? What is the role of influential current global health actors, including the Global Fund for AIDS, Tuberculosis and Malaria, the Gates Foundation and political bodies such as the United Nations?

E) Global health ethics and its values

As is no doubt evident, the complexity of what seems at first to be a simple problem can be overwhelming. There is a need to examine deeply each level and understand how the levels are linked and intertwined. Ethical analysis can assist us in this process. By ethics, we mean understanding how to evaluate different courses of action – and their social consequences – in a given situation (see Chapter 2). Ethics can serve as a lens to understand relationships and power dynamics between different groups, and it can help us discern who benefits and who bears the burdens. Ethics commences with self-reflection, and hence brings to the surface our own motivations for actions, requiring us to look inward (as individuals and collectively as societies) to identify the impetus and consequences of these actions. Global health ethics is about both avoiding the enormous risks of doing harm, and encouraging individuals to do what is best given particular sets of circumstances and constraints. Ethics also requires dialogue and deliberation with others who may or may not share the same guiding motivations. Often, the fundamental principles and missions of individuals and organizations may not be transparent, requiring a disciplined and critical approach to make them more evident.

Most professions require some training in ethics and also have standards and regulations around professional behaviour. Global health ethics does not replace this, but builds on it. An additional focus on the ethics of global health is necessary because the situations and problems encountered may be different from the context in which a trainee or practitioner studies and works (Schwartz et al. 2010). Resources in many communities – in both LMIC and HIC – are limited in various ways. It is important to understand how material contexts change a situation and place a higher priority on, for example, the need to limit waste or to reach the most vulnerable people. There is often a great difference in power and privilege between the provider and recipient of services, particularly within a clinical context. In LMIC, the roles of different actors may be less well defined and there may be less oversight or regulation than in HIC. There may also be cultural differences and diversity in social norms and political beliefs. It is precisely because global health – as noted above – has emerged from a history of colonialism and imperialism that we must be mindful of how this legacy influences relationships between communities and organizations (see Chapter 9). Global health should thus be 'inherently an ethical enterprise' (DeCamp 2011: 92).

Global health ethics draws on classical clinical bioethics, public health ethics and humanitarian ethics (see Chapters 3, 7 and 8) (Pinto and Upshur 2009). It builds on existing codes of professional practice in the health arena, including those issued by the International Council of Nurses (2006), the World Medical Association (2006), the International Federation of Red Cross and Red Crescent Societies (1994) and the Humanitarian Charter (Sphere Project) (2004). Less work has been done within health professional education programs (Crump et al. 2010; DeCamp 2011), and this book aims to address the needs of those in training or who are early in their career.

F) Conclusion

To summarize, global health is an emerging discipline that traces its origins, norms and organizational structure to tropical and colonial medicine and international health, making it highly problematic in that it continues to reproduce the asymmetries of power extant in its predecessors. Notwithstanding its enormous growth, global health remains a contested arena. Ethical analysis creates a space for reflection and deliberation about issues such as social justice, fairness, our professional duties and the duties of others. It is about asking why, interrogating power relations and bringing a critical perspective to all such work. Such analysis must be grounded in the lives of individuals and communities, lest it become an abstract intellectual exercise that does not truly inform global health action (Benatar and Upshur 2011). We believe that global health ethics can assist you in becoming a better practitioner, academic and educator, and that it is crucial to achieving the goal of collectively improving health for all.

References

Anderson, M. et al. (2006) *First Nations, Métis, and Inuit health indicators in Canada.* Background paper for the project 'Action oriented indicators of health and health systems development for Indigenous peoples in Australia, Canada, and New Zealand'.

Arnold, D. (1997) 'The place of "the tropics" in Western medical ideas since 1750', *Tropical Medicine and International Health*, 2(4): 303–13.

Australian Government (2009) *Closing the Gap on Indigenous Disadvantage: The Challenge forAustralia.* Canberra: Australian Government.

Benatar, S. and Upshur, R.E.G. (2011) 'What is global health?', in: Benatar, S. and Brock, G. (eds), *Global Health and Global Health Ethics*. Cambridge & New York: Cambridge University Press.

Berlinguer, G. (1992) 'The interchange of disease and health between the Old and New Worlds', *American Journal of Public Health*, 82(1): 1407–13.

Birn, A.-E. (2006) *Marriage of Convenience: Rockefeller International Health and Revolutionary Mexico*. Rochester: University of Rochester Press.

— (2009) 'Making it politic(al): Closing the Gap in a Generation: Health Equity through Action on the Social Determinants of Health', *Social Medicine*, 4(3): 166–82.

— (2011) 'Remaking international health: refreshing perspectives from Latin America', *Pan American Journal of Public Health*, 30(2): 106–10.

Birn, A.-E., Pillay, Y. and Holtz, T.H. (2009) *Textbook of International Health: Global Health in a Dynamic World*, 3rd edn. New York: Oxford University Press.

Borowy, I. (2009) *Coming to Terms with World Health: The League of Nations Health Organisation 1921–1946*. Frankfurt: Peter Lang–International Academic Publishers.

Bozorgmehr, K. (2010) 'Rethinking the "global" in global health: a dialectic approach', *Globalization and Health*, 6(19).

Brown, T.M., Cueto, M. and Fee, E. (2006) 'The World Health Organization and the transition from "international" to "global" public health', *American Journal of Public Health*, 96(1): 62–72.

Bynum, W. (1993) 'Policing hearts of darkness: aspects of the International Sanitary Conferences', *History and Philosophy of the Life Sciences*, 15(3): 421–34.

Campbell, O., Graham, W.J. and Lancet Maternal Survival Series Steering Group (2006) 'Strategies for reducing maternal mortality: getting on with what works', *Lancet*, 368(9543): 1284–99.

Catalano, R., Goldman-Mellor, S., Saxton, K., Margerison-Zilko, C., Subbaraman, M., LeWinn, K. and Anderson, E. (2011) 'The health effects of economic decline', *Annual Review of Public Health*, 32: 431–50.

Costello, A., Abbas, M., Allen, A., Ball, S., Bell, S., Bellamy, R. et al. (2009) 'Managing the effects of climate change', *Lancet*, 373(9676): 1693–1733.

Crane, J. (2011) 'Scrambling for Africa? Universities and global health', *Lancet*, 377(9775): 1388–90.

Crump, J.A., Sugarman, J. and Working Group on Ethics Guidelines for Global Health Training (WEIGHT) (2010) 'Ethics and best practice guidelines for training experiences in global health', *American Journal of Tropical Medicine and Hygiene*, 83(6): 1178–82.

Cueto, M. (ed.) (1994) *Missionaries of Science: The Rockefeller Foundation and Latin America*. Bloomington: Indiana University Press.

DeCamp, M. (2011) 'Ethical review of global short-term medical volunteerism', *HEC Forum*, 23(2), 91–103.

De Cock, K.M., Lucas, S.B., Mabey, D. and Parry, E. (1995) 'Tropical medicine for the 21st century', *British Medical Journal*, 311(7009): 860–62.

Farmer, P., Drobac, P. and Agoos, Z. (2009) 'Colonial roots of global health: lessons learned for modern humanitarian health', *Harvard College Global Health Review*, 19 September.

Fried, L.P., Bentley, M.E., Buekens, P., Burke, D.S., Frenk, J.J., Klag, M.J. et al. (2010) 'Global health is public health', *Lancet*, 375: 535–37.

Gow, J. (2002) 'The HIV/AIDS epidemic in Africa: implications for U.S. policy', *Health Affairs*, 21(3): 57–69.

Graham, W.J., Fitzmaurice, A.E., Bell, J.S. and Cairns, J.A. (2004) 'The familial technique for linking maternal death with poverty', *Lancet*, 363(9402): 23–7.

Gwatkin, D.R., Rutstein, S., Johnson, K., Suliman, E., Wagstaff, A. and Amouzou, A. (2007) *Socio-economic Differences in Health, Nutrition and Population within Developing Countries: An Overview*. Washington, DC: World Bank.

Harrison, M. (2006) 'Disease, diplomacy and international commerce: the origins of international sanitary regulation in the nineteenth century', *Journal of Global History*, 1: 197–217.

Hutchison, J.F. (1996) *Champions of Charity: War and the Rise of the Red Cross*. Boulder: Westview Press.

Institute of Medicine (1997) *America's Vital Interest in Global Health: Protecting our People, Enhancing our Economy, and Advancing our International Interests*. Washington, DC: National Academy of Sciences.

— (2009) *The U.S. Commitment to Global Health: Recommendations for the Public and Private Sectors*. Washington, DC: National Academies Press.

Jones, G., Steketee, R.W., Black, R.E., Bhutta, Z.A., Morris, S.S. and the Bellagio Child Survival Study Group (2003) 'How many child deaths can we prevent this year?', *Lancet*, 362(9377): 65–71.

Kickbusch, I. (2002) 'Influence and opportunity: reflections on the US role in global public health', *Health Affairs*, 21: 131–41.

Koplan, J.P., Bond, T.C., Merson, M.H., Reddy, K.S., Rodriguez, M.H., Sewankambo, N.K. and Wasserheit, J.N. (2009) 'Towards a common definition of global health', *Lancet*, 373(9679): 1993–95.

Labonté, R., Mohindra, K. and Schrecker, T. (2011) 'The growing impact of globalization for health and public health practice', *Annual Review of Public Health*, 32: 263–83.

Larson, C.P., Haddad, S., Birn, A.-E., Cole, D.C., Labonté, R., Roberts, J.H. et al. (2011) 'Grand Challenges Canada: inappropriate emphasis and missed opportunities in global health research?', *Canadian Journal of Public Health*, 102(2): 149–51.

Macfarlane, S.B., Jacobs, M. and Kaaya, E.E. (2008) 'In the name of global health: trends in academic institutions', *Journal of Public Health Policy*, 29(4): 383–401.

MacLean, S.J. and MacLean, D.R. (2009) 'A "new scramble for Africa": the struggle in sub-Saharan Africa to set the terms of global health', *The Round Table: The Commonwealth Journal of International Affairs*, 98(402): 361–71.

MacLeod, R. and Lewis, M. (eds) (1998) *Disease, Medicine and Empire: Perspectives on Western Medicine and the Experience of European Expansion*. London: Routledge.

McCord, C. and Freeman, H.P. (1990) 'Excess mortality in Harlem', *New England Journal of Medicine*, 322: 173–77.

McCoy, D., Chand, S. and Sridhar, D. (2009) 'Global health funding: how much, where it comes from and where it goes', *Health Policy and Planning*, 24: 407–17.

Navarro, V. (ed.) (1981) *Imperialism, Health and Medicine*, Amityville, NY: Baywood.

Ollila, E. (2005) 'Global health priorities – priorities of the wealthy?', *Globalization and Health*, 1(6).

Packard, R.M. (1997) 'Malaria dreams: postwar visions of health and development in the third world', *Medical Anthropology: Cross-Cultural Studies in Health and Illness*, 17(3): 279–96.

Pinto, A.D. and Upshur, R.E.G. (2009) 'Global health ethics for students', *Developing World Bioethics*, 9(1): 1–10.

Public Health Agency of Canada (2004) *The Social Determinants of Health: An Overview of the Implications for Policy and the Role of the Health Sector*. Ottawa: Public Health Agency of Canada.

Said, E.W. (1979) *Orientalism*. New York: 1st Vintage Books.

Schwartz, L., Sinding, C., Hunt, M., Elit, L., Redwood-Campbell, L., Adelson, N. et al. (2010) 'Ethics in conditions of disaster and deprivation: learning from health workers' narratives', *American Journal of Bioethics – Primary Research*, 1(3), 45–54.

Starfield, B. (2006) 'State of the art in research on equity in health', *Journal of Health Politics, Policy and Law*, 31(1): 11–32.

Stuckler, D., Basu, S., Suhrcke, M., Coutts, A. and McKee, M. (2011) 'Effects of the 2008 recession on health: a first look at European data', *Lancet*, 378(9786): 124–25.

Walt, G. (1993) 'WHO under stress: implications for health policy', *Health Policy*, 24(2): 125–44.

Whitehead, M. (1992) 'The concepts and principles of equity and health', *International Journal of Health Services*, 22(3): 429–45.

Wood, R., Sutton, M., Clark, D., McKeon, A. and Bain, M. (2006) 'Measuring inequalities in health: the case for healthy life expectancy', *Journal of Epidemiology and Community Health*, 60: 1089–92.

WEF (2012) 'World Economic Forum Annual Meeting 2012, Davos–Klosters, Switzerland, 25–29 January'. World Economic Forum. www.weforum.org/events/world-economic-forum-annual- meeting-2012

WHO (2008) *Closing the Gap in a Generation: Health Equity through Action on the Social Determinants of Health*. Final Report of the Commission on Social Determinants of Health. Geneva: World Health Organization.

— (2011a) *World Health Statistics 2011*. Geneva: World Health Organization.

— (2011b) 'Millennium Development Goals: Progress towards the Health-related Millennium Development Goals'. Geneva: World Health Organization. www.who.int/mediacentre/factsheets/fs290/en/index.html

— (2011c) 'Rio Political Declaration on Social Determinants of Health', in: *World Conference on Social Determinants of Health, 19–21 October 2011*. Geneva: World Health Organization.

— (2012) 'Commission on Macroeconomics and Health (CMH)'. Geneva: World Health Organization. www.who.int/trade/glossary/story008/en/index.html

2 Ethics and global health

Ross E.G. Upshur, Solomon Benatar and
Andrew D. Pinto

Objectives

- To introduce the range of ethical concepts and approaches to ethical analysis required in global health work
- To outline frameworks of principles that have been applied within clinical medicine, public health and global health
- To develop the concepts of **solidarity** and **social justice** as principles to guide global health work

A) Introduction

In Chapter 1, the history and origins of global health were outlined. Consideration of ethical issues at the level of global health requires first a clear understanding of the early twenty-first-century context in which global health challenges need to be addressed. Three fundamental issues call for particular attention: resource disparities and power relationships; the role of globalized/liberalized trade; and global media and information. These frame our discussion on ethical principles and ethical reasoning.

Resource disparities and power relationships

The world is characterized by grotesquely wide disparities in health and in access to the social, economic, political and health care channels that could be used to reverse widening trends. Access to power and how power is used lies at the heart of the problem of global health disparities. Power is usually thought of as the hard power of the military or other forms of coercive force, and this is not totally unrealistic. However, given the relationship between wealth – here modestly defined as access to basic needs for human development and a flourishing life – and health, the fact that a small proportion of people determine how the global economy operates and who will benefit, and at whose expense, makes it clear that economic power outstrips military power in determining the global distribution and burden of health and disease. Although these two forms of power are not unlinked, the long-known adverse role of the currently structured global political economy has been either denied or obfuscated by those in economic power who are covertly deeply implicated in causing human poverty and misery on a massive scale (Benatar 2005). Additional evidence for this is provided by the extent of human harm that has flowed from the recently unfolding global economic crisis (Benatar et al. 2011b).

Consider for a moment the impact on Americans. Since the economic crisis began in 2008, $5 trillion has been lost by Americans in pensions and savings. Approximately $15 trillion was lost in the value of homes by 2010, with 10,000 homes entering foreclosure each day (13 million expected by 2014). In 2009, 1.4 million Americans filed for bankruptcy, an increase of 32 per cent from 2008. Moreover, medical bankruptcies accounted for 60 per cent, and 75 per cent of the latter were filed by people with health insurance. Personal debt amounting to 65 per cent of income in 1980 increased to 125 per cent of income by February 2009 (DeGraw 2010).

Over the past century, annual income distribution to the top 1 per cent of people in the USA fell from 25 per cent in 1925 to 10 per cent in 1970 (a period of economic and industrial growth and expansion of the middle class), then rose back to 25 per cent by 2008 under the impact of the neoliberal policies that geared economic growth to the benefit of the wealthy (Sachs 2011). Disparities in wealth are thus almost as wide within the USA as they are across the globe, and these are accompanied by wide disparities in health. Even in the USA, there is food insecurity among children who suffer from preventable hunger, and the fact that 9 million American children lack health insurance points to the potential for preventing premature suffering and death. These examples, which highlight the impact of fiscal trends on the value accorded to the health and lives of children in the wealthiest and most privatized health market (the United States), typify the global redistribution of resources during the past half century, with disastrous effect on those who live below subsistence levels elsewhere in the world (Benatar et al. 2011b).

For example, a combination of low economic growth, rising unemployment and rising food prices in 2009 pushed up the number of chronically hungry people globally from 850 million to over a billion. Between 2003 and 2006, maize increased in price by more than 50 per cent of its average price, and by 2008 rice prices were 100 per cent higher than they were in 2003. Such increases, together with the immediate effects of higher energy prices, have pushed more than 100 million people back into poverty and ill health.

The role of globalized/liberalized trade

Since the later 1970s, the global political economy and trade rules have been transformed by the ideas and practices associated with the ideology of neoliberalism (Gill and Bakker 2011). Disciplinary neoliberalism, the dominant discourse of political economy since 1970, serves libertarian ideas, institutions, political forces and policies to deepen the power of capital and to shape patterns of global economic and social development. The New Constitutionalism, which is the political–juridical counterpart to disciplinary neoliberalism, creates treaties and codifies new rights and freedoms for firms and investors. These are manifest in laws, rules and regulations, of which intellectual property rights is one example (Gill and Bakker 2011)

Globalization and global trade, driven by these polices, have been promoted under the assumption that 'globalization is good for the poor'. However, the basis for this claim, and the implications of trade policies for social equity, have been heavily criticized, most specifically in relation to regulations affecting food and a range of health matters, including trade in pharmaceuticals, the availability of vaccines in epidemics and the international recruitment of health professionals.

Another result of such policies has been the exploitation of labor, nature and social processes, with particularly adverse effects on health, welfare, education, and other social support structures such as pensions. Health care, like food and oil, is increasingly becoming a commodity distributed through the power of an emerging new hybrid of public and private health care institutions that are extensively governed by world market forces. The privatization of goods and of services that serve the common good has impaired the ability to reproduce the caring social institutions (health care, education and other public social services) on which good societies depend in order for their citizens to have the best opportunity to reach their human potential and to flourish. Pandering to the endless entitlements of those at the top of the economic pyramid has been undertaken at the cost of the health and wellbeing of the majority. As a consequence, almost 50 per cent of the world's population lives on less than $3 per day and on about 3 per cent of annual global product.

Global media and information

The media, in an era of rapid communication, disseminate vast amounts of information, with increasing and often underappreciated influence on how we conceptualize the world around us, what we believe and how we behave. The extent to which the media control how the public thinks and acts (as exemplified by marketing strategies and the fear agenda actively promoted since 9/11, allowing the acceptance of stringent new security processes that undermine hard-won liberties) has deflected attention from garnering widespread support for the available constructive means of improving the health and wellbeing of billions of people worldwide in the twenty-first century.

All these influences on global health call for ethical arguments to effect change.

B) Ethical concepts and ethical reasoning

You may be outraged about the existence of health inequities and the fact that it seems all lives are not considered of equal value. In doing something about this, you probably want to do the right thing. What is considered to be the right thing, in many given contexts, is neither self-evident nor necessarily universally shared. In fact, it is more than likely that there may be conflict regarding how different individuals, communities and organizations conceptualize the 'right' thing.

Ethics, in the broadest sense, embraces the range of methods used to critically analyze, interpret and evaluate the variety of ways in which humans interact with each other. In the most general terms, ethics seeks to provide an account of how humans, as agents, assign and evaluate the worth of persons, organizations, their actions and their consequences. From a more philosophical perspective, ethics engages in appraising the range of arguments offered to determine the rightness or wrongness of actions and policies, and reflects upon the praiseworthiness or blameworthiness of actors and organizations, and the justification for such judgments. Many of the concepts informing such thinking emerge from culture with origins in a variety of traditions, both religious and secular. Although there is a great deal of diversity in how people think about moral issues, there are no societies without a concept of what is right and wrong. Ethics is distinct from the law in that it addresses issues related to interpersonal duties and obligations that are not regulated or compelled by external authority.

Historically, ethical reflection and ethical reasoning have embraced a wide range of accounts of how these activities take place. Within the Western tradition, numerous attempts have been made to systematize approaches to ethics in the form of major ethical theories. Some of these are based entirely on secular considerations, others have their origin in theology or faith-based communities. In this section we introduce some major themes in ethical analysis. We do so by very briefly outlining the nature of ethical theory, and distinguishing ethical frameworks from ethical theories. Some general considerations on defining and understanding ethical reasoning are also developed. This is followed by a general discussion on the major schools of thought that have animated ethical thinking, and a description of some of the major ethical frameworks used in health care. We then discuss some of the features that make global health ethics distinct from clinical and public health ethics.

In an introductory text, it is impossible to discuss such a rich, complex and varied literature in detail. While this book does not intend to replace the education in bioethics that is a required training component of health professionals and of other students considering work in global health, it is recommended for use within such courses. It is our contention that ethical reasoning skills, including an ability to identify and analyze the value issues that may be latent and undisclosed in the many contexts relevant to global health, are essential and fundamental skills for global health practitioners. There is no substitute for engaging in reflection and dialogue, a skill that improves with practice.

C) Ethical theory and applied ethics

It is important to recognize the distinction between ethical theories and applied ethics. Ethical theories aspire to provide a comprehensive, consistent and defensible normative account of moral activity. Historically, the field of ethical theory has been the domain of philosophy.

An ethical theory must achieve several goals: it must set out to explain and justify, in a unifying manner, a wide range of considerations including the nature of morality, and the principles or concepts and criteria by which human actions are evaluated. This often includes a systematic and nuanced account of the positive reasons why a particular theory is more capable than rival theories of providing accounts of moral issues. Hence the argumentation found in works of moral theory is often dense, technical and exhaustive with respect to dealing with potential counterarguments to the position articulated. It is important to distinguish descriptive from normative accounts of ethics (see Box 2.1).

Box 2.1: Descriptive and normative ethics

Descriptive ethics relates to accounts of how humans actually behave in the world. It has a strong empirical dimension as it derives from descriptions of how moral values play out in determining what is right or wrong in various communities. It is thus dependent on reliable empirical observations of how humans assess the rightness and wrongness of their actions. In the field of global health, observations come from academic disciplines such as epidemiology, sociology, anthropology, law, political science and psychology.

Normative ethics focuses on a different dimension of human activity. Rather than describing what is actually done, normative ethics considers the question of what we should (or ought to) do in order to bring about 'ethical states' of affairs rationally.

Predominant ethical theories in the Western tradition

Universalist approaches

Schools of thought can be considered universalist when the theory argues that a universal and objective criterion or test can be applied to human actions to adjudicate its rightness or wrongness. The Western tradition has been influenced and shaped by three dominant universalist approaches: deontological, consequentialist and virtue based.

i) Deontological
Deontological approaches are typified by arguments that focus on the moral worth of actions, that is, that certain acts are intrinsically right or wrong; and on rational analysis of such acts. It is important to note that, according to this approach, ethical acts are appraised largely independently of consciously calculated potential consequences that follow from them. This is not to deny that outcomes in general shape what we consider to be right and wrong actions.

The foremost account of a deontological approach is found in the work of the philosopher Immanuel Kant. Kant's moral theory is based on the requirement that moral values be stated as universal laws. The abstract and general formulation of the law-like structure of moral statements is the categorical imperative. The categorical imperative states that one should act only 'on that maxim which you can at the same time will to be a universal law'. These laws are to command assent by all rational agents capable of acting freely upon them. The requirements are universal in the sense that they do not depend on anything in the empirical world for their justification. That is, the entire structure of laws is established a priori.

Kantianism is influential in that it establishes important conditions for the treatment of moral agents. They must be treated as ends in themselves and not as means to an end. This notion is influential in doctrines such as human rights, and informs standards for human subject protection in global health research. It is the ethical theory most closely aligned with accounts of human dignity and inherent worth.

ii) Consequentialist
Consequentialist theories view the rightness or wrongness of actions in terms of the consequences that result from the action. The classical formulation of consequentialism is utilitarianism, where the best action is that which creates the greatest good for the greatest number. Classic utilitarianism is 'hedonistic' in nature, in that it argues that happiness and pleasure are the consequences to be maximized. There are many variations on consequentialist theories, and they are prominent in modern health ethics. Consequentialist theories are associated with economic analyses such as cost–benefit and cost–effectiveness analysis, and with such tools as disability-adjusted life years (DALYs), quality-adjusted life years (QALYs) and other outcome measures that are relied on in making public health policies, as distinct from decisions about individual patients.

iii) Virtue based
Rather than focusing on acts or their consequences, virtue-based approaches examine the qualities, characteristics and habitual actions of human agents. Thus they focus on the appraisal of character in the context of action. Virtue theories focus on such manifest qualities as courage, humility, caring and wisdom. In more broad community applications, virtue theory discusses the qualities and characteristics of communities that give rise to virtuous citizens.

Relativist and non-cognitivist approaches

These are accounts of ethics arguing that morality is not based on objective, universal and rational considerations, and that it cannot be so based. There are two principal schools of thought in this regard: relativism and non-cognitivism.

i) Relativism
Relativism holds that standards of determining the rightness and wrongness of actions are related to and hold only for those who participate in a particular culture and community. They admit to no overarching universal claim that all humans should follow.

ii) Non-cognitivist
Non-cognitivist accounts hold that ethical statements have no truth-value whatsoever, and are merely the expression of emotions and personal preferences.

Religion-based approaches

Religious ethics cannot be ignored in considerations of individual or population health, as many communities in the world base their institutions and practices in accord with religious principles. In each of the three predominantly monotheistic religions, Islam, Judaism and Christianity, ethical appraisal consists of the application of sacred texts and generations of commentary and reflection on the ethical problem at issue. Casuistry is the term used to describe this 'looking back' to precedents for guidance. Each of these major religions has several variations of practice and interpretation of sacred texts (indicating significant within-religion disagreement). In religious ethics, fidelity to the dictates of faith, as indicated by the sacred texts, is of critical importance. There are many points of agreement, but also significant areas of disagreement between these religions. There are numerous other faiths, such as Hinduism and Buddhism, that influence thinking and popular ideas relevant to health care. It is imperative for practitioners to be aware of and respectful of religious practices and how certain health activities may be interpreted in light of revealed religion. While respecting individuals' religious beliefs when they are choosing for themselves, there is a need to be cautious that in the public realm some religious perspectives are not privileged over others.

Applied ethics: the concept of ethical frameworks

There is considerable variation and complexity in how we can make sense of distinguishing which human actions are ethical or moral. In order to facilitate the application of complex theory to practice, the field of applied ethics has developed approaches intended to guide practitioners.

There are a variety of ways of doing this. One way is through the creation and application of frameworks. In applied ethics, it is recognized that certain theories have attractive features in certain circumstances, but seem strained in application to all cases that may be encountered. They should be viewed as resources that aid in the understanding of ethical problems and in decision-making. In essence, such theories provide a set of diverse perspectives on how best to understand an ethical issue.

Frameworks have been proposed as a way of making this complex landscape tractable, to aid in the analysis of ethical issues and to guide reflection and decision-making. When there is reluctance to engage with the finer points of moral theory, frameworks can be used as pragmatic tools to aid decision-making. Frameworks can be very useful because they attempt to capture what is relevant to decision-making in a particular area of practice. They help to simplify and make explicit factors relevant to a decision. However, they can also be problematic if they are applied blindly (Dawson 2010). It is important that the framework is relevant to the particular area under discussion, as a framework can yield a poor answer if it does not capture all the factors relevant for a particular decision.

As global health is an immensely complex field, there is a need for a multiplicity of perspectives to be understood and balanced. Understanding ethical issues in global health requires inter-professional, trans-disciplinary and transcultural understanding.

Classical bioethics has explored many ethical issues at the individual level. In most health care professional training, ethics is taught in terms of the need to consider four key principles: autonomy, beneficence, non-maleficence and justice. This classic formulation from the work of Thomas Beauchamp and James Childress (2005) has been quite useful and influential in ethics pedagogy, and still serves a very useful purpose. It attempts to reconcile the two main strands of thought in the Western tradition: deontology and consequentialism.

A recently evolving discourse on public health ethics provides some additional principles and frameworks for thinking and arguing about public health dilemmas, where there is a need to weigh and balance the rights of individuals against the common good. This expanded discourse, like the feminist approach, provides additional values for consideration and appropriate frameworks with which to do so. Public health ethics, in many ways, provides a grounding for global health ethics in that it addresses issues related to common goods, and employs concepts that focus on collective responsibilities and mutuality (Dawson and Verweij 2007; Nixon et al. 2008).

No one theory or framework will describe and analyze the same issue in the same way. Hence familiarity, experience and practice are required. Frameworks aim to assist in understanding the various dimensions involved in decision-making and acting, but they will not supply all the answers, and individual judgment is still required.

Ethical reasoning and argumentation: a suggested approach

Ethical theories and ethical frameworks will direct practitioners to the substantive issues informing an analysis of an ethical dilemma. Reasoning should be approached systematically and in a fair and dispassionate manner.

One first consideration is fair explication of the various positions at issue. This requires close reading and accurate knowledge of the relevant facts. It is important to understand the distinction between factual claims and normative claims (see Box 2.2). Then one must be able to assess the types of claims that are being made and the type of argument that is being stated. This requires sorting out the various factual and moral claims that are at issue. Box 2.3 provides a systematic approach to analyzing an ethical issue.

Box 2.2: Facts and values

Most philosophical accounts of ethics tend to make a sharp distinction between facts (usually construed as statements from science or empirical observations) and values (desirable but perhaps not realized states of affairs in the life world). What is factual tends, for the most part, to reflect or contain descriptions of states of affairs. Values, on the other hand, reflect normative evaluations about what ought to be the case. One issue arising from this is the gap between what is the case (descriptive facts) and what ought to be the case (how things should change towards, or be, for a more ethical state of affairs). Many have argued that it is impossible to derive an 'ought' from an 'is', that is, a description of a state of affairs in no way entails a prescription about how to change that state of affairs in the world. While the distinction between facts and values ('isness' and 'oughtness') plays a significant role in the evolution and history of moral philosophy, these tend to interpenetrate considerably, particularly in the sphere of applied health ethics.

Box 2.3: A systematic approach to ethical reasoning*

1   What are the morally relevant facts in the case?

2   How/on what basis are they morally relevant? That is, what moral principles, theories or concepts underlie your determination of what is morally relevant? What are your underlying implicit and explicit values?

3   How would you prioritize the ethical issues inherent in the case – which are the most morally relevant? As above, what underlies your decision (principles, values, etc.)?

4   How would you deal with possible conflicting ethical considerations?

5   What bearing does moral psychology have? For example, can you discern the intent that lies behind your moral reasoning?

6   Once you have worked through the above, have your views changed in terms of what is morally relevant about the case?

7   How would you discuss/dialogue with the community involved about your views on the case?

8   How does your role/organizational-specific authority (e.g. legal, medical, professional) impact on the way in which you adjudicate the case? What bearing might this have on how you approach the above, particularly number 7?

9   Are there any particular global issues that arise in the analysis? If so, what are the morally salient aspects of this global dimension? Are these issues arising at the personal, health system, population and/or global levels?

*Adapted from Richardson (2007)

Argumentation consists of the ordering of reasons that lead to a well-justified conclusion. Premises are statements that, taken together, demonstrate logical connection, consistency and coherence. Much argumentation to which we are exposed in everyday life is at a very low level of sophistication, and in fact is not argumentation, but simple assertion. It often consists of simple declarations that 'X is wrong' or 'X is unethical' without supporting reasoning grounded on some more basic principle. We must avoid simple assertion without supporting reasons. Many ethical arguments concern the weighing and balancing of seemingly conflicting principles or goods that we seek to attain. One common strategy is simply to argue for that which one believes. This often results in not taking counterarguments seriously or acknowledging uncertainty or limitations in one's own perspective. Ideally, we should strive to take seriously all candidate arguments, positive and negative, and seek out and rebut any potential objections to the perspective we are taking. When we approach moral reasoning in this manner, we are taking a fair and measured approach and enhancing reciprocal awareness and respect for others.

Concepts of justice

Justice is a fundamental concept in ethics, and accounts of justice date back to antiquity. In the most fundamental sense, justice is concerned with issues related to equality and fairness. As Aristotle noted, justice requires that we treat equal persons equally and unequal persons unequally. Theories of justice have their basis in deontological, consequentialist, virtue theory and feminist traditions. The concept of social justice is discussed in detail later in this chapter.

The most relevant considerations of justice in global health relate to various theories of distributive justice. Distributive justice consists in the study of the normative principles guiding how the benefits and burdens of economic activity are best allocated. Health is included in the scope of these allocative decisions.

There is a range of competing theories of how best to allocate resources. These theories are rooted in fundamental conceptions of how humans and societies are ideally to be constituted (Lamont and Favor 2007). The most commonly held perspectives will be very briefly sketched out. Most of these theories look at justice from within an established legitimate nation state. There is an immense volume of literature on this topic, and readers are advised to consult the suggested reading list at the end of this chapter for further exploration of the topic. Commonly held views include the following.

- **Egalitarianism:** that every person is owed the same level of benefits, and this is based on concepts of equality of persons.
- **Welfare:** that the welfare of people is the paramount norm. All other principles of distribution are secondary to the maximization of welfare.
- **Desert-based theories:** that benefits and burdens should be distributed on the basis of the actions of persons and societies that create the benefits.
- **Libertarianism:** that benefits and burdens should be distributed according to the function of free markets.

The work of John Rawls has been particularly influential in modern theories of justice (Rawls 1999). For Rawls, justice is fundamentally related to liberty, such as the right to basic freedoms and equality of opportunity. Differences in terms of these fundamental liberties, such as inequalities of opportunity, should exist only insofar as they are of benefit to those with least advantage.

Much writing in global justice seeks to overcome some of the limitations of the application of theories of justice to within nation states alone. However, this is contentious and depends on whether there are good arguments for obligations to others beyond state borders based on considerations of justice. Thomas Pogge is one of the most influential theorists in this area. He argues that severe poverty is the most pressing issue of global justice, and that as well as a positive responsibility to alleviate poverty, there is a 'negative responsibility to stop imposing the existing global order and to prevent and mitigate the harms it continually causes for the world's poorest populations' (Pogge 2001: 22).

D) Key dimensions of global health ethics

What is global health ethics?

Hunter and Dawson (2011) provide an account of the ways in which global health ethics can be regarded as a distinct field of inquiry. In essence, global health ethics requires an account for why we should care about the fate and existence of others, often quite remote from us. This is particularly challenging in times of economic hardship, when it may seem self-evident to be concerned with one's own locality.

Global health ethics can be understood in a geographic sense in that it addresses issues that have broad spatial concern, such as climate change. This view of global health ethics is, however, likely to be too limited when applied to the types of ethical issues that require analysis. A content view of global health ethics is one that addresses specific ethical issues such as research ethics and global health equity. This account is limited by a lack of systematic coherence.

Hunter and Dawson (2011) argue that global health ethics should be regarded as a substantive normative endeavour in its own right. They outline three arguments in favour of this substantive account: the beneficence argument; considerations of justice and harm; and cosmopolitanism.

The argument for beneficence regards global health inequalities as 'morally objectionable in and of themselves, because they hold that differences in outcomes need to be morally justified and that there does not seem to be a justification in this case' (Hunter and Dawson 2011: 79). This is best expressed in Peter Singer's claim that 'If it is in our power to do or prevent something bad from happening, without thereby sacrificing anything of comparable moral importance, we ought, morally, to do it' (Singer 1972 quoted in Hunter and Dawson 2011: 80). Arguments from beneficence provide a 'prima facie reason to accept substantive global health ethics' (Hunter and Dawson 2011: 80).

The argument from justice and harm is based on Thomas Pogge's work, which argues that global obligations are rooted in negative duties not to harm others and to make reparations when others have been harmed. As shown in Chapter 1, the history of exploitation and domination by many nations has led to the current state of global economic and health inequalities, many of which are perpetuated by current global governance structures.

Cosmopolitanism indicates that we are citizens of a globalized world, and further argues that moral considerations are not based solely on the prerogatives of membership in a particular nation state, culture or ethnic group. Cosmopolitanism requires us to have a global frame of mind when addressing issues in global health.

Frameworks in global health

As noted, frameworks are limited in what they can offer – providing only a way to view an issue or a problem. However, they may assist students and practitioners to understand the morality of global health, the 'norms about right and wrong human conduct' in this value-laden field. Values evolve over time and in relation to their contexts and thus we should ask, what values should guide our work at this moment in global health?

Benatar et al. (2011a) have outlined a framework that argues for global health ethics as a rationale for mutual caring. They identify seven values required as a basis for global health ethics:

- respect for all human life
- human rights, responsibilities (duties) and needs – broadly considered
- equity
- freedom (freedom from 'want' as well as freedom 'to do')
- democracy (in a participatory sense)
- environmental ethics
- solidarity.

They argue that none of these principles can stand alone to provide an overarching account of the values of global health ethics, and that solidarity is the most important value of all.

They also propose a framework for transformational approaches:

- developing a global state of mind
- promoting long-term self-interest
- striking a balance between optimism and pessimism
- developing capacity (to be independent)
- achieving widespread access to public goods.

Putting these transformational approaches into practice requires systematic reflection and engagement with communities locally and globally. Chapter 4 on human rights and Chapter 11 on advocacy explore how these transformational approaches can take place.

In the remainder of this chapter, we build upon this framework and one that we have proposed previously: humility, introspection, social justice and solidarity (Pinto and Upshur 2009), adding depth and broadening its applicability. Humility and introspection are addressed in Chapter 3. We will place particular focus on social justice and solidarity.

E) Social justice and global health

Social justice has been cited frequently as a core value that underpins global health. It is named in the strategic plans of academic centres of global health, in the vision statements of non-governmental organizations, and in the policy papers of key bodies such as the World Health Organization (WHO). This can be traced to a long history of identifying social justice as central to public health (Beauchamp 1976), and even as *the* foundational moral justification for interventions at the population level (Powers and Faden 2006).

Yet diverse definitions exist about what social justice is and how we can achieve it (Braveman 2006). A recent WHO discussion paper focuses on looking at *how societies are organized*, and on social justice as *promoting the 'common good'* to which all in the society are expected to contribute (WHO 2011). Further, promoting social justice is to *uphold basic human rights and equitable access to resources*. Similarly, Krieger has defined social justice – particularly within a research context – as about *understanding who benefits and who is harmed* by certain policies or decisions (Krieger 2001). Many others reinforce the concept that social justice is about *ensuring a minimum standard of living, redistributing societal resources* and achieving an *egalitarian society*. Public health's 'dream' of a society without the current unequal distribution of health and its determinants – health inequities – is therefore closely tied to the aims of social justice (Beauchamp 1976).

To understand how this applies to global health, we focus on three interrelated areas: the drive to reduce health inequities; distributional justice; and the health of marginalized populations (Bayoumi and Guta 2012).

Reducing health inequities – unjust and unfair differences in health outcomes between groups that are linked to the rules that govern society (Dahlgren and Whitehead 2007) – is central to the mandate of global health (see Chapter 1). Identifying such differences between communities requires forethought when designing epidemiological surveys and posing research questions; when considering how to analyze the data collected; and when disseminating the results (see Chapter 8). However, describing inequities is not sufficient to achieve social justice. Work to reduce inequities requires innovative solutions that address root causes in the social determinants of health (Muntaner et al. 2009).

Social justice as applied to global health is also concerned with distributional justice, meaning identifying and rectifying differences in who benefits from global resources. Are those who have equal need receiving equal treatment (horizontal equity)? And are those with a great need for resources receiving more than those with lesser needs (vertical equity)? Within social justice, we look beyond the classic interpretation of justice in the allocation of healthcare services at the individual level to the distribution of wealth, opportunities for education and employment, and access to healthy environments at the community, country and international levels. Often, such calls for distributional justice are tied to the concept of human rights, or claims that citizens can make on state powers (see Chapter 4). Concrete proposals for redistributing resources at the global level have included novel taxes on financial transactions (e.g. Tobin tax), carbon taxes, and exemptions to trade regulations (e.g. TRIPS exemptions). Calls for alternatives to global neoliberalism, which exemplifies market justice rather than social justice, have been built on a recognition that the growing gap between the rich and the poor is directly related to our current economic and political system (Benatar et al. 2011b; Labonté and Schrecker 2011).

Many global health commentators have called for a focus on the most marginalized – those who exist at the metaphorical margins of our society. As Farmer notes, global health should be based on a preferential option for the most disadvantaged (Farmer

2003). This is a third part of unpacking social justice, as the marginalization of groups and communities occurs due to discrimination, racism, and the continuation of historical injustices and unfair policies that benefit some at the expense of others. This has encouraged some to use equity lenses or health equity impact assessment to draw attention to how interventions can sometimes worsen health differences between groups. For example, when a health promotion campaign leads to improved uptake of a positive behavior amongst the better-educated, wealthier segment of a population.

Western medicine – embedded within its historical and economic context – has often been reluctant to engage in such issues as are deemed 'too political'. Critical examination of society, understanding overt and covert power relations, and identifying means to reduce inequities are underdeveloped, with few exceptions (Waitzkin et al. 2001). A learned helplessness around social justice sets in, particularly if a clinician is trained to see herself as working in isolation from others. We contend that social justice is a societal-level challenge and requires multiple and related social movements (see Box 2.4). Political problems call for political solutions, not technical solutions (Bayoumi and Guta 2012). Throughout, community consultation must be taken seriously, with action being directed at creating solutions that will actually benefit the most marginalized.

Box 2.4: Social movements

Social movements are distinct social processes where actors engage in collective action, and are characterized by involvement in conflictual relations with clearly identified opponents, dense informal networks, and a shared and distinctive collective identity (Porta and Diani 2006). Social movements relate to the central functions of public health, particularly that of promoting healthy communities. When organized around perceived threats to health, they can play a crucial role as advocates for change (Nathanson 1999).

Social movements emerge from the intersection of the personal, the collective and the historical. They are impacted by societal norms and attitudes, political opposition and the media, and do not emerge fully formed. Often, many small groups federate around a core idea to achieve collective action around a common mission. Ultimately, they are composed of people who become activated, who get politicized and in turn policitize others (Eyerman 1989).

Social movements develop out of certain contexts, typically a mix of four dimensions:

- changes in basic conditions of life that produce discontent
- change in the beliefs and values used to respond to life circumstances
- change in the capacity to act collectively
- change in the opportunity for successful action (e.g. weakness of the opposition, support from powerful allies, success of other social movements) (Oberschall 1993).

There is a long history of health social movements, defined as 'collective challenges to medical policy, public health policy and politics, belief systems, research and practice which include an array of formal and informal organisations, supporters, networks of cooperation and media' (Brown et al. 2004: 52). Much of the history of modern public health was intimately tied to social movements, particularly struggles around the social determinants of health (Krieger and Birn 1998). The theory and values of health promotion emphasize the importance of community mobilization and action (e.g. from the Ottawa Charter: 'At the heart of this process is the empowerment of communities – their ownership and control of their own endeavours and destinies. Community development draws on existing human and material resources in the community to enhance self-help and social support, and to develop flexible systems for strengthening public participation in and direction of health matters') (WHO 1986). Health social movements make an impact by producing changes in the health and public health system, by stimulating change in science and the selection of certain hypotheses to test, and by changing institutions that shape health, including funding organizations and policy-makers (Brown et al. 2004).

An exemplar of a global health social movement has been the struggle to achieve universal access to HIV/AIDS medications. In high-income countries, the demand for treatment was built on the growing gay rights social movement, the community that was hardest hit by the unfolding epidemic. In low-income countries, particularly sub-Saharan Africa, people living with HIV/AIDS and allies used legal mechanisms such as court challenges around the right to health to oppose patent restrictions on medications. In concert with a broad, global social movement that targeted pharmaceutical companies, these efforts provoked governments to take action (Forman 2008). Of note, the failure to fully link these two social movements has resulted in the current disparity in access that we see between North and South (see Chapter 4).

F) Solidarity and global health

A second powerful value to bring to global health work is solidarity, which we posit begins within the practice of humility, reflexivity and introspection – situating oneself in the world (see Chapter 3). It is intimately related to the operationalization of social justice. Solidarity is a sociological term first brought into academic usage in 1893 by Durkheim, who distinguished mechanical solidarity from organic solidarity. Mechanical solidarity existed when people related to one another based on similarities, such as their common religion, tribe or ethnicity. This similar identity produced a 'collective consciousness' and people were motivated to work together towards a common goal: the benefit of the group. In more modern societies, people relate to one another based on the division of labor, and hence their differences. Organic solidarity is developed through mutual interdependence and a reliance on others, with an emphasis on the individual (Durkheim 1984).

This history is important, as Durkheim uses 'solidarity' in an overall analysis of society from a political economy perspective, focusing on power relations and the relationship of power to resources and institutions. The term retained its political connotations during the twentieth century, and was famously used as the name of the Polish union that brought about democratic change in the 1980s. Pope John Paul II, a strong supporter of the anti-Communist movement in Poland, used the term in his encyclical of 1987, *Sollicitudo Rei Socialis*. He called for a realization of the Christian duty of solidarity, developing the idea as embracing a sense of universality, interdependence, and that 'people are realizing that they are linked together by a common destiny, which is to be constructed together' (Ioannes Paulus 1987). Solidarity continues to be the name of several trade unions in Europe and North America, and the title of many labor publications. We define solidarity here as relationships arising from common responsibilities and interests, as between members of a group or between people, enacted by individuals as they align their goals and values with those of the community in which they are working. Such relationships allow approaches to be built that permit us to relate authentically and for mutual benefit across distances.

Solidarity has been cited as key to addressing common threats, such as pandemics and climate change (Brody and Avery 2009). It is also a value to guide public health programs to reach marginalized communities (Ruger 2009). However, solidarity is perhaps most relevant to global health as an alternative to traditional, charity-based approaches. As Galeano wrote: 'Unlike solidarity, which is horizontal and takes place between equals, charity is top-down, humiliating those who receive it and never challenging the implicit power relations' (Galeano 1998). Charity, or 'helping', leads to the disempowerment of community leaders, systems and infrastructure, the degradation of autonomy and a loss of self-determination, and increased community vulnerability to external exploitation. There is increasing concern that external influence and pressure within communities receiving aid programs in the name of helping may be left worse off than prior to a helping intervention (Yamin 2011).

Solidarity exists when citizens of the community are mobilized, when capacity building of local organizations and strengthened links within civil society occurs, and when attempts are made to bridge power imbalances between the wealthy and the poor. It is an active and ongoing process. Barriers to solidarity include having conflicting views of health and its determinants, and not recognizing and focusing on power and resource differentials. Facilitators of solidarity include developing and maintaining deep, honest relationships and open, purposeful communication, and being explicit about who bears the benefits and who bears the burden of any global health initiative.

What would a partnership based in solidarity look like? Ideally, this partnership would be crafted from building blocks of equality and attempts at mutual understanding. In a solidarity approach, as individual change-makers we must clarify our motivations and interrogate power relationships within the relationships we form. The goal of such a partnership would lead to positive, lasting change coming from inside a community. Ideally, this would be a pioneering, creative experience. This partnership would provide a container where members of a community could feel socially safe to make authentic, thoughtful contributions to a community problem.

A relationship based in solidarity, where two people – perhaps from different backgrounds, different communities – are working for a common goal, would encourage them both to be innovative and creative in approaches to problems. It would create the right environment for the right conversations, where the right questions are asked. It would provide a space where each party could bring their unique skills and contributions to the table for them to be used to serve the team in an environment of respect.

Solidarity is put into action in global health through various means. Humanitarian medical organizations such as Doctors Without Borders employ witnessing (*témoignage*) as a means of expressing solidarity with individuals and populations whose health has been put at risk owing to war, civil strife or natural and human-made disasters. Building meaningful partnerships and collaborations with communities is also an effective means of bringing solidarity from an abstract principle to a lived engagement (see Chapter 9).

G) Conclusion

Certainly, global health ethics is in its infancy. Medical ethics has evolved since the 1970s and transformed the relationship between physicians and patients through a focus on individuals. The emergence of new infectious diseases, and the challenges of setting priorities in the face of escalating demands and limited resources, have stimulated a renewed discourse on public health ethics in which considerations of the common good require greater attention and justification. In the face of a 'complex organic crisis' characterized by multiple overlapping crises that threaten the health of all globally, there is now a need for yet another ambitious discourse on global health ethics. Whether or not we consider this to be intellectually viable, the need to narrow wide and widening injustices in health cannot be ignored (Hunter and Dawson 2011). We have attempted to show here some of the directions in which such thinking needs to advance.

While it can be objected that global health ethics is yet another example of domination from the North, we contend that there has been increasing evidence of perspectives from low- and middle-income countries taking similar critical stances (see Chapter 10). Much more needs to be done to advance a global dialogue, particularly efforts to minimize obstacles to the dissemination of views. Some may feel that discussions about ethics do not translate into practical action to improve health. We argue that any effort within global health rests on some form of ethical commitment, and that these commitments are often tacit and under-conceptualized. Attention to the ethical dimensions of interventions holds the possibility of altering them in fundamental ways. Finally, we have argued that global health ethics entails more than merely attending to issues in distributive justice. As noted above, looking towards the transformational capacity of ethics may help bring about a global state of mind that can lead to more equitable health outcomes.

References

Bayoumi, A.M. and Guta, A. (2012) 'Values and social epidemiological research', in: O'Campo, P. and Dunn, J.R. (eds), *Rethinking Social Epidemiology*. Dordrecht: Springer.

Beauchamp, D.E. (1976) 'Public health as social justice', *Inquiry*, 13(1): 3–14.

Beauchamp, T.L. and Childress, J.F. (2001) *Principles of Biomedical Ethics*. New York: Oxford University Press.

Benatar, S.R. (2005) 'Moral imagination: the missing component in global health', *PLoS Medicine*, 2(12): e400.

Benatar, S.R., Daar, A. and Singer, P.A. (2011a) 'Global health ethics: the rationale for mutual caring', in: Benatar, S.R. and Brock, G. (eds), *Global Health and Global Health Ethics*. Cambridge: Cambridge University Press, 129–40.

Benatar, S.R., Gill, S. and Bakker, I. (2011b) 'Global health and the global economic crisis', *American Journal of Public Health*, 101(4): 646–53.

Braveman, P. (2006) 'Health disparities and health equity: concepts and measurement', *Annual Review of Public Health*, 27: 167–94.

Brody, H. and Avery, E.N. (2009) 'Medicine's duty to treat pandemic illness: solidarity and vulnerability', *Hastings Center Report*, 39(1): 40–8.

Brown, P. et al. (2004) 'Embodied health movements: new approaches to social movements in health', *Sociology of Health & Illness*, 26(1): 50–80.

Dahlgren, G. and Whitehead, M. (2007) *Policies and Strategies to Promote Social Equity in Health: Background Document to WHO – Strategy Paper for Europe*. Stockholm: Institute for Future Studies.

Dawson, A. (2010) 'Theory and practice in public health ethics: a complex relationship', in: Peckham, S. and Hann, A. (eds), *Public Health Ethics and Practice*. Bristol: The Policy Press.

Dawson, A. and Verweij, M. (2007) *Ethics, Prevention and Public Health*. New York: Oxford University Press.

DeGraw, D. (2010) 'The economic elite have engineered an extraordinary coup, threatening the very existence of the middle class', *AlterNet*, www.alternet.org/story/145667

Durkheim, E. (1984) *The Division of Labour in Society*. New York: Macmillan.

Eyerman, R. (1989) 'Social movements: between history and sociology', *Theory and Society*, 18(4): 531–45.

Farmer, P. (2003) *Pathologies of Power: Health, Human Rights and the New War on the Poor*. Berkeley: University of California Press.

Forman, L. (2008) '"Rights" and wrongs: what utility for the right to health in reforming trade rules on medicines?', *Health and Human Rights*, 10(2): 37–52.

Galeano, E. (1998) *Upside Down: A Primer for the Looking-Glass World*. New York: Picador.

Gill, S. and Bakker, I.C. (2011) 'The global crisis and global health', in: Benatar, S.R. and Brock, G. (eds), *Global Health and Global Health Ethics*. Cambridge: Cambridge University Press.

Hunter, D. and Dawson, A. (2011) 'Is there a need for global health ethics? For and against', in: Benatar, S.R. and Brock, G. (eds), *Global Health and Global Health Ethics*. Cambridge: Cambridge University Press, 77–88.

Ioannes Paulus PP II (1987) 'Sollicitudo rei socialis', *The Vatican*, www.vatican.va/holy_father/john_paul_ii/encyclicals/documents/hf_jp-ii_enc_30121987_sollicitudo-rei-socialis_en.html

Krieger, N. (2001) 'A glossary for social epidemiology', *Journal of Epidemiology and Community Health*, 55(10): 693–700.

Krieger, N. and Birn, A-E. (1998) 'A vision of social justice as the foundation of public health: commemorating 150 years of the Spirit of 1848', *American Journal of Public Health*, 88(11): 1603–6.

Labonté, R. and Schrecker, T. (2011) 'The state of global health in a radically unequal world: patterns and prospects', in: Benatar, S.R. and Brock, G. (eds), *Global Health and Global Health Ethics*. Cambridge: Cambridge University Press.

Lamont, J. and Favor, C. (2007) 'Distributive justice', *Stanford Encyclopedia of Philosophy*, http://plato.stanford.edu/archives/fall2008/entries/justice-distributive

Muntaner, C. et al. (2009) 'Against unjust global distribution of power and money: The report of the WHO commission on the social determinants of health: global inequality and the future of public health policy', *Journal of Public Health Policy*, 30: 163–75.

Nathanson, C.A. (1999) 'Social movements as catalysts for policy change: the case of smoking and guns', *Journal of Health Politics, Policy and Law*, 24(3): 421–88.

Nixon, S.A. et al. (2008) 'Public health ethics', in: Bailey, T.M., Caulfield, T. and Ries, N.M. (eds), *Public Health Law & Policy in Canada*, 2nd edn. Toronto: Lexis Nexis Butterworths, 37–59.

Oberschall, A. (1993) *Social Movements: Ideologies, Interests and Identities*. London: Transaction.

Pinto, A.D. and Upshur, R.E.G. (2009) 'Global health ethics for students', *Developing World Bioethics*, 9: 1–10.

Pogge, T. (2001) 'Priorities of global justice', *Metaphilosophy*, 32(1/2): 6–24.

Porta, D. and Diani, M. (2006) *Social Movements: An Introduction*, 2nd edn. Oxford: Blackwell Publishing.

Powers, M. and Faden, R. (2006) *Social Justice: The Moral Foundations of Public Health and Health Policy*. New York: Oxford University Press.

Rawls, J. (1999) *A Theory of Justice*. Cambridge: Harvard University Press.

Richardson, H. (2007) 'Moral reasoning', *Stanford Encyclopedia of Philosophy*, http://plato.stanford.edu/entries/reasoning-moral

Ruger, J.P. (2009) 'Global health justice', *Public Health Ethics*, 2(3): 261–75.

Sachs, J. (2011) *The Price of Civilization: Economics & Ethics after the Fall*. Toronto: Random House.

Waitzkin, H. et al. (2001) 'Social medicine then and now: lessons from Latin America', *American Journal of Public Health*, 91(10): 1592–601.

WHO (1986) 'Ottawa Charter for Health Promotion', First International Conference on Health Promotion, 21 November 1986. Geneva: World Health Organization.

— (2011) 'Discussion paper: Closing the gap: policy into practice on social determinants of health', World Conference on Social Determinants of Health, Rio de Janeiro, 19–21 October. Geneva: World Health Organization.

Yamin, A.E. (2011) 'Our place in the world: conceptualizing obligations beyond borders in human rights-based approaches to health', *Health and Human Rights*, 12(1): 3–14.

Further resources

Books

Benatar, S.R. and Brock, G. (eds) (2011) *Global Health and Global Health Ethics*. Cambridge: Cambridge University Press.

Singer, P.A. and Viens, A. (eds) (2008) *The Cambridge Book of Bioethics*. Cambridge: Cambridge University Press.

Declarations and codes of ethics

UNESCO Universal Declaration on Bioethics and Human Rights:
www.unesco.org/new/en/social-and-human-sciences/themes/bioethics/bioethics-and-human-rights

World Medical Association International Code of Medical Ethics:
www.wma.net/en/30publications/10policies/c8

International Council of Nurses, Code of Ethics for Nurses:
www.icn.ch/about-icn/code-of-ethics-for-nurses

3 Approaching global health as a learner

Malika Sharma and Kelly Anderson

Objectives

- To articulate questions that bind us together as global health learners
- To identify shared elements in the cycle of global health education
- To encourage **introspection** and **humility** in global health learning

---

Case study 3.1

A family medicine residency in an inner-city setting

Ram recently graduated from medical school in a high-income country (HIC). Beforehand, he spent two years working in northern India with community health workers. About to start a residency in family medicine, he wonders how to reconcile his previous experiences with a medical career that incorporates global health. Ram's medical training and undergraduate degree in development studies have influenced his understanding of global health. He sees himself traveling to a low-income country and working with local non-governmental organizations, both practicing medicine and working in program development and evaluation. He starts a family medicine residency in an inner-city setting and finds that most of his patients are on social assistance and many are dealing with chronic pain, addictions or mental health issues. Although he struggles with ways to make a meaningful impact, he enjoys his work and sees a connection between what he is doing and the ideas and principles of global health.

Case study 3.2

An internship at an HIV service organization in Rwanda

Mili recently completed a Master's in Public Health in a HIC. She has an interest in community-based research and works on a study being carried out locally with recent immigrants and refugees on barriers to care. She finds meaning in this work and wonders if this is an example of global health. Her interests lead her to consider working in Sub-Saharan Africa, and ultimately she accepts a four-month funded internship working at an HIV service organization in Rwanda. Upon arrival, she has difficulty communicating in French with her colleagues and learns little of the local language. Throughout her time there, she finds herself socializing mostly with other expatriates. She begins work on several initiatives, but they do not progress beyond the proposal stage. Upon her return home, she wonders what she should have done differently, and begins to reflect on what her motivations were for going in the first place.

A) Introduction

What are the enduring solutions to creating healthy and resilient communities (Wheatley and Frieze 2011)? Those asking this question are global health learners. They are students, trainees, activists, artists, academics, practitioners, researchers, teachers, policy-makers and politicians. Some are new learners with varying degrees of interest; others are already experts in their field. Yet all ask questions such as: Where do we fit within global health? How can the right to health be achieved for all? What obstacles lie in the way? How do we ensure our work reflects solidarity and not charity (see Chapter 2)?

This chapter explores these questions and examines how learners go about finding answers. This process is shaped by an individual's context, motivations and knowledge, all learners have similar questions and experiences. To understand the global health learning cycle, we outline four common steps (Figure 3.1), similar to the model described by Arnold et al. (1991) and discussed elsewhere (see Chapter 12).

Step 1 is about **orientation**. Learners start to ask themselves and others fundamental questions, and are shaped by the answers they find. Step 2 is the **visceral experience,** where the learner is put into a global health setting and is confronted by logistical, moral and ethical questions. Step 3 involves **introspection** and honest **self-reflection** about one's motivations, power and privilege and the limits of individual efforts. Step 4 entails **relearning global health,** where learners begin to appreciate the dynamic nature of global health. Humility is the hallmark of this stage. A clearer sense of how to engage in global health as a career is developed through this cycle.

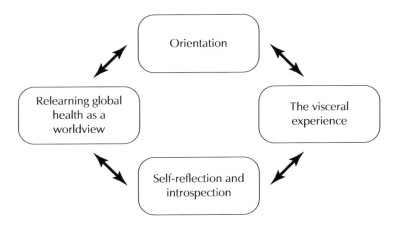

Figure 3.1 The global health learning cycle

B) The global health learning cycle

Step 1: Orientation

Learners begin the cycle through hearing about 'global health' and becoming interested in learning more. What is global health (see Chapter 1)? How is it different from public health, international health or tropical medicine? Where does global health take place? Who practices global health? Who are leaders in this field and what do they do? Is engaging in research, education or community-based field work all forms of global health?

The array of ideas and concepts that fall under the umbrella of global health can be daunting, but common themes of health equity, human rights and both individual and population-level interventions emerge (Koplan et al. 2009). Today, most learners accept that global health is not simply about working in low- and middle-income countries (LMIC), but can involve working in high-income countries (HIC) with indigenous communities, the homeless in urban settings and those without legal status. Indeed, a learner's mentors and personal learning experiences will continue to reinforce the link between marginalization and global health (Jarvis-Selinger et al. 2008).

Finally, learners in HIC will begin to contend with the problematic history of global health (see Chapter 1) and what this means today in terms of an ongoing connection to foreign policy and 'corporate colonialism' (Anonymous 2004). As learners grow in their political and historical understanding of global health, they may begin to question whether global health initiatives can lead to deepening inequalities and further exploitation (Benatar 1998). Unfortunately, many may ignore such thoughts in order to justify the experiences they want to have.

Step 2: The visceral experience

A common assumption of the global health learner is that she/he must go 'abroad' to gain experience. Learners often embark on international electives, service learning or volunteer positions, bringing them face-to-face with the issues they have only so far read or heard about. Most often these experiences occur in LMIC. In 2009, 43.2 per cent of graduating American medical students had participated in an international elective during their undergraduate medical training (AAMC 2010).

There are well-documented educational benefits for learners pursuing international experiences in low-resource areas: a positive influence on diagnostic skills, positive attitudinal changes, increased knowledge of tropical diseases, and increased consideration of career choices within primary care and underserved populations (Thompson et al. 2003; Dowell and Merrylees 2009). However, the risks of global health electives are less frequently considered. Can unprepared and inexperienced trainees face ethical challenges and cause harm? Are there safety risks to themselves and to the communities in which they study (Pinto and Upshur 2009)?

Bishop and Litch (2000) highlight the risk of medical tourism, defined as 'travel to a developing region with a brief opportunity to practice medicine on local community members' (Bishop and Litch 2000: 1017). They ask: 'If as a doctor you cannot resist the lure of medical tourism and insist on the casual or opportunistic treating of local residents, consider whether you are treating the patient for your own good or for theirs, and whether your actions may actually do more harm than good' (Bishop and Litch 2000: 1017). Medical tourism can undermine existing health care structures and cause unexpected harm, and this is true for all health professionals. Many learners find themselves in clinical situations with little supervision, making decisions that they are inadequately qualified to make. Shah and Wu (2008) describe an elective student's realization that he may have sent a child home with a life-threatening condition because of his junior level of training. This same trainee described stories of his colleagues performing unsupervised procedures far beyond their level of expertise while on international electives. Many international experiences involve trainees from resource-rich countries traveling to countries and institutions in the global South, with no remuneration to the host institution. These students may also take precious teaching time from local trainees. Other risks for learners who are ill-prepared include culture shock, missed learning opportunities, inappropriate levels of responsibility and a lack of cultural sensitivity, which could potentially cause harm in the host community (Shah and Wu 2008).

Unfortunately, most students are ill-prepared for these experiences. In a 2005–06 survey of Canadian medical schools, almost half did not provide adequate oversight or supervision to students on elective (Izadnegahdar et al. 2008). There remains a relative paucity of pre-departure training, which is variable across organizations (Anderson et al. 2012). This is all the more concerning as trainees are participating in these experiences earlier and earlier in their training (Shah and Wu 2008).

The desire for a visceral experience leads to another discomforting question: is there a desire to intervene in the lives of others to make them 'better'? If so, who has taught us this need, and on what assumptions is this based? Global health learners with an urge to change the systems and cultures they encounter, without a full understanding of context, culture and history, are a risk to the communities they are visiting. Their enthusiasm, although rooted in good intention, is often missing a critical understanding of historical and cultural norms, as well as the inherent strengths and belief systems of a community. Anthropologist Wade Davis notes about non-Western communities 'these peoples are not failed attempts at being modern, quaint and colourful, destined to fade away by natural law...these are dynamic living peoples being driven out of existence by identifiable forces' (Davis 2009: 167). Are visiting learners a small part of these forces? Can hands-on global health experiences teach us to learn from the communities we visit instead of trying to help while imposing Northern values and expectations? Illich (1968) declares 'If you insist on working with the poor, if this is your vocation, then at least work among the poor who can tell you to go to hell.'

Alternatives to an international experience do exist. Local communities may introduce the learner to questions of power, politics and social determinants of health, without some of the risks described. We may be more linguistically and culturally prepared to start our hands-on global health learning at home, and more capable of asking questions about motivations, impact and risks of harm when working in our own backyard.

Step 3: Introspection

It is often the visceral elective experience, and an accompanying sense that 'something is not quite right', that pushes the learner to start to identify their own power and privilege. Learners may also realize that their motivations are not as altruistic as originally imagined, and may question whether their experience was potentially harmful to the very population they aimed to serve.

The learner may begin to question the basic premise that those in the global North are in a position to help those in the South, along with the faulty assumption that 'some care is better than none'. This awareness may prevent a trainee from working above their level of training and causing harm. It may lead to greater respect for the knowledge and skills of local providers. It may even lead a trainee to forgo pursuing any further experiences or deferring them until later in her/his training. This humility may be combined with questions about entitlement. What are our privileges, and from where do they spring (Pinto and Upshur 2009)? Do we have the right to travel to another country to study and work there? Why do internationally trained physicians and trainees face numerous barriers to practicing, even for brief periods, within HIC? The learner must recognize that 'medical training in a developed world context does not translate to competence in all settings' (Pinto and Upshur 2009: 7). Humility is essential to undermining the neocolonialism that can characterize North–South relationships.

There may also be a re-examination of motivations. Philpott (2010) categorizes these motivations into those we would rather suppress, those we can tolerate, and those to which we aspire. A willingness to acknowledge less palatable or admirable motivations, such as 'the desire for professional escapades to punctuate an otherwise dreary career' (Philpott 2010: 231), does not make them any less real, but may help cultivate humility and transform our global health learning journey. Were we influenced by the hero myth? Often, global health 'heroes' share a common story: they were called to adventure, underwent trials and tribulations in a foreign land, and returned home changed (Rosenzweig 1996). This myth becomes even more entrenched when we return home to loved ones, who tell us how proud they are that we want to 'save the world'. Dagi (1988) turns the problem of 'physician as hero' on its head, using this paradigm instead to suggest that physicians are called to address the broader determinants of health and social injustice. Here, the physician is a 'paragon of virtue', willing to assume risks, pursue knowledge and act to improve society as a whole. However, Dagi (1988) recognizes the dangers inherent in this hero mythology, which can lead to 'a savior mentality; a sense of invulnerability; a sense of entitlement and social mandate; and a highly paternalistic approach to interactions with patients and with the institutions of society' (Dagi 1988: 57).

Learners may question why they felt they were called to serve in this hero role. Certainly, humanitarian celebrities play a role by inspiring us, and at times demonstrating social justice in action and speaking 'truth to power' by virtue of their position. Does seeking our own heroism build into our motivations around global health work? How does the quest for awards and accolades fall into our plans? Learners must question this impulse and be cognizant of the impact it can have on the people they are aiming to serve, who risk becoming mere subjects in our hero's tale.

Another danger of the hero myth is the 'danger of the single story' (Adichie 2009). When we create and narrate a story to ourselves and others about our global health experiences, '[we] create stereotypes, and the problem with stereotypes is not that they are untrue, but that they are incomplete. They make one story become the only story.' Any singular story can dispossess or disempower, as it is often impossible to relay a story with objective cultural and historical context. When using a cultural competency-based approach to understand their global health experience, trainees may actually further 'other' certain communities. By focusing too heavily on ethno-cultural characteristics, rather than an understanding of class, geography and political factors as key determinants of a patient's health, they may fail to understand the complexities of identity that involve race, ethnicity, class, gender and sexual orientation. Rather, this approach simplifies patients or groups into one overarching identity (e.g. African) (Wear 2003).

Students should reflect on how and whether they are implicitly participating in this simplification, or telling of 'a single story', and whether they are failing to 'connect the idea of diversity with the underlying core concept of social justice in health care' (Wear 2003). Adichie (2009) adds, however, that 'stories can...be used to empower and to humanize...stories can break the dignity of a people, but stories can also repair that broken dignity'. In our examination of our experiences and their consequences, we must consider how we use our stories and what unexpected effects telling those stories may have. Does the way we internally examine and communicate our experience build or break stereotypes, empower or disempower, expand or contract the ability of those around us to understand the scope of global health?

Finally, how have we been changed by our global health experience? Learners may find the immense luxury in the global North unsettling or disturbing after witnessing extreme poverty in low-income settings. We may find the applause from family and friends jarring, when recognizing that the task of addressing health inequities is far larger than anything we could have tackled on our own. We may return home incensed by the injustice that we have witnessed. We may feel compelled to enact change in some way, or alternatively may feel defeated by our seeming inability to change the circumstances in our host communities. We may feel a sense of discomfort in sharing our experience, sensing that we are in some ways putting the poverty of others on display. Razack (2007) refers to this peculiar consumption of the pain and suffering as 'stealing the pain of others', and compels us to recognize our economic, missionary and even moral complicity, and to question the ways in which we may use other people's suffering to validate things we believe about ourselves, such as our strong humanitarian impulses or caring natures. This reflection is even more pressing in the digital era, where blogs and online photo essays may provide catharsis for the writer, but may also exploit the grief, suffering and poverty of their patients (Bhan 2005).

This complex process of introspection is meant to be reflexive as well as constant. Trainees are encouraged to ask themselves a number of questions before proceeding on a global health elective (see Box 3.1). However, they will invariably revisit these questions and ask new ones after their global health experience. This iterative process allows learners to cultivate global health as a worldview and, ideally, develop a pattern of lifelong learning.

Box 3.1: Questions for students prior to global health work (adapted from Pinto and Upshur 2009)

- Why do I hope to do this work?
- What are my objectives (personal and structural, short- and long-term)?
- What are the benefits and who will receive them?
- What are the costs and who will bear them?
- What do I need to do to prepare for my experience, both practical and personal?
- Is it fair to impose my presence on a community when power imbalance, language or cultural difference may impede my ability to understand how welcome or useful I am?
- Can I address or prepare for these issues before my departure?
- What are the specific weaknesses in my plan?
- Is the work feasible, cost-effective, necessary, focused and justified?
- Will it work to undermine disparity or actually contribute to it?
- What do I hope to bring back to my community and with whom will I share it with?
- How will I assess my impact, both subjectively and objectively?
- Where will I get my feedback from?

Step 4: Relearning global health as a worldview

Continual learning is an ongoing process rather than a discrete point in the learner's trajectory. We come to realize that our experiences, analysis and self-reflection will continually alter our perceptions of what global health actually means. We discover that global health is more a way of looking at health and inequalities, rather than a static field of study or work. We may question whether simple answers exist at all. This openness to discomfort can help us discover new ways of community-building, and learn more deeply about belief systems that differ from our own. Over time, we develop a clearer sense of how we may pursue a career in global health and try to find mentors who will foster our vision, as well as institutions that will support us in those goals.

To develop this expansive analysis of global health, learners often turn to further education. Although an institution's global health curriculum may be strong, the learner must remain critical of its underlying philosophies. Many Northern institutions are enthusiastically forming partnerships with Southern universities. The speed of these developments may not allow for adequate time to address ethical concerns and develop sustainable relationships (Crane 2011). When choosing an institution within which to study, it may be incumbent on the learner to ensure she is part of a thoughtful, collaborative partnership (Chapter 9).

Inspiration is critical at all stages of the learning journey as we seek answers to uncomfortable questions and sometimes face disillusionment. Surrounding ourselves with peers and community members who share and expand our ways of thinking can be an incredible source of support. Cultivating mentorship is another central aspect to creating a community of practice. The right mentor can provide insight and inspiration, and encourage learners at pivotal and paradigm-shifting moments in their careers (Anderson and Anspacher 2011). How can mentees actively seek out effective but more informal mentorship? Students must be perseverant and proactive in their search, including setting up meetings with potential mentors. They must foster the characteristics of an effective mentee: passion to succeed, proactivity and willingness to learn (Jackson et al. 2003). Similarly, effective mentees prepare for meetings with their mentors, provide a suggested outline for each discussion, and complete assigned tasks (Sambunjak et al. 2010).

Lastly, daily experiences can inform our ways of thinking. Does our daily work create opportunities to engage in local global health sustainably? How might we build upon these opportunities? Developing global health as a worldview means finding the applicability of global health in all of these avenues.

C) Conclusion

The global health learning cycle (Figure 3.1) is meant to represent the dynamic, flexible nature of the learner's path. Many learners move from initial questioning to self-reflection without the need for a visceral experience. By understanding and articulating these various stages, we have a platform to examine some of the ethical challenges faced by global health learners from the North.

It is essential to create a space and process for self-reflection as part of this journey, allowing us to understand the potential risks and benefits associated with global health experiences in low-resource areas. Our ultimate goal is not to discourage global health work by trainees, but rather to encourage trainees to engage in their learning in the most ethical, sustainable and just way possible.

Case resolution 3.1

Ram enjoys his inner-city family medicine residency, but struggles with the recognition that most of his patients live below the poverty line. He realizes that his medical training takes him only so far when dealing with the complex issues many of his patients face. Early in his residency, he has the opportunity to travel to Tanzania on a short-term medical elective, but declines, recognizing he is not yet comfortable to work independently in that type of setting. After completing his residency, he decides to explore family medicine opportunities in northern Canada, having realized that global health is about marginalized communities regardless of location. With the permission of a few of his patients, he begins writing narrative pieces that highlight the social determinants of health. He is confident that he can continue to weave global health concepts into his work locally.

Case resolution 3.2

Mili continues to grapple with the difficult questions she began to explore upon her return home from Rwanda. She realizes that she was nowhere near as useful to the community as she had anticipated, and even wonders if the money spent on her position would have better served her host community in other ways. She regrets her relatively little interaction with local colleagues there, and feels that four months was too short to understand the dynamics of the local environment and institution. However, she decides to persevere with international HIV work, joining a large non-governmental organization in the field of monitoring and evaluation. While living in Montreal, she travels regularly to countries in West Africa to learn from local programs and attend conferences. Although she still sees ethical challenges in her work, she feels supported by her organization and is ready to continue asking these difficult questions to ensure she acts as ethically and responsibly as possible.

References

Adichie, C. (2009) 'The danger of a single story' [TED talk], http://blog.ted.com/2009/10/07/the_danger_of_a

Anderson, K. and Anspacher, M. (2011) 'Mentorship in global health education', in: Chase, J. and Evert, J. (eds), *Global Health Training in Graduate Medical Education: A Guidebook*, 2nd edn. San Francisco: Global Health Education Consortium.

Anderson, K. et al. (2012) 'Are we there yet? Preparing Canadian medical students for global health electives', *Academic Medicine*, 87(2): 206–9.

Anonymous (2004) 'Tropical medicine: a brittle tool of the new imperialism', *Lancet*, 363(9415): 1087.

Arnold, R. et al. (1991) *Educating for a Change*. Toronto: Between the Lines.

AAMC (2010) *2010 GQ Medical School Graduation Questionnaire: All Schools Summary Report Final*. Washington, DC: Association of American Medical Colleges, https://www.aamc.org/download/140716/data/2010_gq_all_schools.pdf

Benatar, S.R. (1998) 'Imperialism, research ethics and global health', *Journal of Medical Ethics*, 24(4): 221–22.

Bhan, A. (2005) 'Should health professionals allow reporters inside hospitals and clinics at times of natural disasters?', *PLoS Medicine*, 2(6): 471–73.

Bishop, R. and Litch, J.A. (2000) 'Medical tourism can do harm', *British Medical Journal*, 320(7240): 1017.

Crane, J. (2011) 'Scrambling for Africa? Universities and global health', *Lancet*, 377(9775): 1388–90.

Dagi, T.F. (1988) 'Physicians and obligatory social activism', *Journal of Medical Humanities and Bioethics*, 9(1): 50–59.

Davis, W. (2009) *The Wayfinders: Why Ancient Wisdom Matters in the Modern World*. Toronto: House of Anansi Press.

Dowell, J. and Merrylees, N. (2009) 'Electives: isn't it time for a change?', *Medical Education*, 43(2): 121–26.

Illich, I. (1968) 'To hell with good intentions', in: *Conference on Inter-American Student Projects (CIASP), Cuernavaca, Mexico, 20 April 1968*.

Izadnegahdar, R. et al. (2008) 'Global health in Canadian medical education: current practices and opportunities', *Academic Medicine*, 83(2): 192–98.

Jackson, V. et al. (2003). 'Having the "right chemistry": a qualitative study of mentoring in academic medicine', *Academic Medicine*, 28(3): 328–34.

Jarvis-Selinger, S. et al. (2008) 'Social accountability in action: university–community collaboration in the development of an interprofessional Aboriginal health elective', *Journal of Interprofessional Care*, 22(S1): 61–72.

Koplan, J.P. et al. (2009) 'Towards a common definition of global health', *Lancet*, 373(9679): 1993–95.

Philpott, J. (2010) 'Training for a global state of mind', *Virtual Mentor*, 12(3): 231–36.

Pinto, A.D. and Upshur, R.E.G. (2009) 'Global health ethics for students', *Developing World Bioethics*, 9(1): 1–10.

Razack, S.H. (2007) 'Stealing the pain of others: reflections on Canadian humanitarian responses', *Review of Education, Pedagogy, and Cultural Studies*, 29(4): 375–94.

Rosenzweig, S. (1996) 'The physician as hero', *Academic Emergency Medicine*, 3(6): 650.

Sambunjak, D., Straus, S. and Marusic, A. (2010) 'A systematic review of qualitative research on the meaning and characteristics of mentoring in academic medicine', *Journal of General Internal Medicine*, 25(1): 72–78.

Shah, S. and Wu, T. (2008) 'The medical student global health experience: professionalism and ethical implications', *Journal of Medical Ethics*, 34(5): 375–78.

Thompson, M.J. et al. (2003) 'Educational effects of international health electives on US and Canadian medical students and residents: a literature review', *Academic Medicine*, 78(3): 342–47.

Wear, D. (2003) 'Insurgent multiculturalism: rethinking how and why we teach culture in medical education', *Academic Medicine*, 78(6): 549–54.

Wheatley, M. and Frieze, D. (2011) *Walk Out Walk On: A Learning Journey into Communities Daring to Live the Future Now*. San Francisco: Berrett-Koehler.

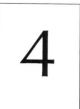

4 Human rights discourse within global health ethics

Lisa Forman and Stephanie Nixon

Objectives

- To provide an overview of international human rights law, particularly the right to health
- To explore the potential contribution of human rights to the achievement of global health equity
- To explore intersections between human rights and global health ethics

A) Introduction

Despite earlier iterations of rights (including the 1776 US Declaration of Independence and the 1789 French Declaration of the Rights of Man), the impetus for the modern development of human rights emerged from the mass violations of the two world wars (Henkin 1990). In 1945, the United Nations (UN) was created, in part to reaffirm faith in "fundamental human rights, in the dignity and worth of the human person, in the equal rights of men and women and of nations large and small" (United Nations 1945: 2). The 1948 *Universal Declaration of Human Rights* was the first explicit human rights instrument of the contemporary system of international human rights law, articulating a broad range of rights to be protected in pursuance of the core human rights values of inherent dignity and equal rights (United Nations 1948). International human rights law recognizes several categories of rights, including *civil and political rights* (including rights to vote, to be free from torture, to have equality before the law, and to have free expression, movement and association) *and economic, social and cultural rights* (including rights to social security, work, education and participation in cultural life). Despite these categories, within international human rights law, all human rights are understood to be indivisible, interrelated and interdependent (United Nations 1993).

Since 1948, these rights have been developed and expanded in multiple human rights treaties, resolutions and declarations, necessitating the development of a comprehensive set of international institutions to monitor and interpret these rights, and prompting the development of regional human rights systems in Africa, the Americas and Europe. These developments have seen human rights become the fastest-growing field in international law (Mutua 2001), with international human rights viewed as having become "constitutive elements of modern and 'civilized' statehood" (Risse et al. 1999: 234).

B) The right to health

The right to health has been protected in international law since the inception of the UN. The 1946 *Constitution of the World Health Organization* recognizes enjoyment of the highest attainable standard of health as a fundamental right of every human being without distinction, and recognizes that governments are responsible "for the health of their peoples which can be fulfilled only by the provision of adequate health and social measures" (WHO 1948: 2). The 1948 *Universal Declaration of Human Rights* recognizes every person's right to a standard of living adequate for her/his health and wellbeing, which includes medical care (United Nations 1948). The 1966 *International Covenant on Economic, Social and Cultural Rights* (ICESCR) contains the most authoritative codification of this right, where state parties recognize everyone's right to the enjoyment of the highest attainable standard of health and agree to take a number of steps to achieve this (United Nations 1966). Subsequently, numerous other international instruments have protected rights to health for specific populations, including racial minorities, women, children, migrant workers and people with disabilities (United Nations 1965, 1979, 1989; UN General Assembly 2007). In addition, each of the regional human rights systems contains treaties with health rights (Council of Europe 1961; African Union 1981; United Nations 1988).

Yet the right to health had little political or social impact until fairly recently. A major development came in 2000, when the UN Committee on Economic, Social and Cultural Rights issued General Comment 14 (UNCESCR 2000), which significantly advanced clarity regarding the scope and content of the right to health and the entitlements it confers on rights-holders, and the corresponding duties it places on states and the international community. The Comment defines this right not only to include people's ability to access adequate, acceptable and good quality health care, but to also access the underlying determinants of health such as food, housing, access to water and adequate sanitation, safe working conditions and a healthy environment (UNCESCR 2000). General Comment 14 specifies state duties corresponding to entitlements under this right, including minimum core duties with which states must comply irrespective of resources, and duties to respect, protect and fulfill access to adequate, affordable health and health care more generally (UNCESCR 2000).

At the international level, the right to health has similarly been advanced through the work of a UN-appointed Special Rapporteur on the right to the highest attainable standard of physical and mental health. The Special Rapporteur's work has further developed the normative content of this right, as well as monitoring accountability for realization of this right by states and other actors. For example, the Special Rapporteur has undertaken missions to multiple countries (including Peru, Uganda, Israel, Lebanon, Colombia, India, Sweden, Australia and Guatemala) as well as to international organizations and non-state actors whose mandates impact on the right to health (including the World Trade Organization, World Bank, International Monetary Fund and GlaxoSmithKline). In addition, the Special Rapporteur has expanded the scope of the right to health by defining pharmaceutical companies' responsibilities in relation to access to medicines (UNHRC 2008). The Special Rapporteur also submits annual reports focusing on issues of particular relevance to the right to health such as poverty, international trade and health systems (OHCHR 2010).

The prominence of this right has similarly been aided through the development of a health and human rights movement globally (Hunt 2006; Beyrer and Pizer 2007; Gruskin et al. 2007; Farmer 2008), emerging from the thesis advanced by Jonathan Mann that human rights and health are in an inextricable relationship (Mann et al. 1999). As a result of the growing health and human rights movement, human rights are now widely seen as essential components of health-practitioner education across a range of disciplines (United Nations 1993; Consortium for Health and Human Rights 1998; International Council of Nurses 1998; World Medical Association 1999; Rodriguez-Garcia and Akhter 2000), with curricula adopted globally at schools of public health, medicine, law and policy studies (Harvard School of Public Health, n.d.).

Nonetheless, the limitations of international human rights law and the right to health must be acknowledged. This body of law is largely applicable to states and deals weakly with the human rights duties of corporations or international organizations. Furthermore, it deals primarily with a state's responsibilities to its own population. These and other controversies provide important context for this chapter's discussion of the contribution of the right to health to global health ethics; for understanding possible institutional and structural factors contributing to its non-realization; and for identifying areas of research required to strengthen the legal and ethical framework relating to global health.

C) Human rights and global health

Human rights and the right to health make a distinctive contribution to efforts to achieve global health equity, through (1) the normative specificity of the right to health and its legally binding nature, (2) its rhetorical impact and potentially to empower rights-holders, (3) accountability mechanisms such as UN country reporting, litigation and advocacy, and (4) the growing adoption of rights-based approaches to health (Forman 2011).

There is growing clarity in international human rights law regarding government duties towards health within instruments such as General Comment 14. The elaboration of these duties provides specificity to governments in fulfilling their population health responsibilities. The duties also provide legal support for rights-based claims in a variety of formats, including advocacy, litigation and UN complaints.

The use of rights rhetoric has the potential to shift health claims from appeals to charity and compassion, to demands based in legally binding duties and justice. A paradigm shift of this nature would see domestic and global policy-makers viewing health not simply as superfluous component of budgetary allocations, but as an area implicating binding legal and moral duties. Rights may also have a transformative impact on the rights-holder, by empowering people to make social and political claims backed with the force of law, and by ensuring that the minimal conditions for individual life and health are met, whether in the form of medicines or housing.

Human rights can also contribute to the achievement of global health equity through the use of international, regional and domestic accountability mechanisms associated with the enforcement of human rights. While most human rights treaties allow individual complaints to be lodged against state parties alleging the violation of treaty rights, there is a dearth of international mechanisms in relation to the right to health. Domestic litigation remains a primary accountability tool in most regions, albeit that its effective use is contingent on a number of factors, including the existence of independent judiciaries. The past decade has seen an exponential rise in right to health litigation globally, including in low- and middle-income countries (Hogerzeil et al. 2006; Yamin and Gloppen 2011). These cases have focused on a wide range of issues, such as access to health services, discriminatory labour practices and various aspects of the basic determinants of health (Gloppen 2008).

The 2002 South African case on perinatal HIV transmission is one such example. In this case, social groups used international and constitutional protections of the rights to health and life to file a case before the Constitutional Court, claiming access to medicine to prevent mother-to-child transmission (MTCT) of HIV (Constitutional Court of South Africa 2002). In its decision, the Court ordered the establishment of a national perinatal program. In South Africa today, a national MTCT programme provides medicines in over 96 per cent of government clinics (Statistics South Africa 2010). Similarly, successful litigation in India and Latin America illustrates how respect for, and promotion of, human rights can lead to improved access to health care as well as increased budgetary allocations to health (Singh et al. 2007; Gloppen 2008).

Rights can also work more systematically to advance health equity than the intermittent incidence and narrow ambit of litigation or issue-based advocacy. Rights-based approaches seek to operationalize the concepts and standards of human rights and offer guidance to policy and programs seeking health equity. They mandate the incorporation of core human rights principles such as non-discrimination, participation and accountability, demand a focus on the poor and marginalized, and require explicit reference to international human rights instruments (Forman and Bomze 2012). One example is a right to health impact assessment which focuses on the implications of policies on the realization of the right to health, and explicitly adopting standards on the right to health drawn from international human rights law (Hunt and MacNaughton 2006). Such tools not only offer the potential to ensure better realization of the right to health, but also may offer procedures for ensuring that governmental actions in other domains, such as trade and commerce, do not unreasonably restrict individuals' right to health (Forman and Bomze 2012).

D) How global health ethics advances human rights

Whereas the section above has considered the contributions of human rights to global health, we now reflect on links to global health *ethics*. We argue that the two fields are synergistic and their contributions taken together stand to offer greater weight than either alone (Nixon and Forman 2008). Nonetheless we acknowledge that there are rare instances where the interests of the two fields may be viewed as in conflict.

A useful starting point is to examine the ethical underpinnings of human rights. At the root of human rights is respect for the worth and equal value of every human life, which may also be framed as the ethical principle of respect for dignity. This focused ethical foundation means that there are aspects of the field of global health ethics that do not fall within the purview of human rights. For instance, global health ethics may include arguments based on compensatory justice to articulate moral obligations of states to address a problem that their own past actions served to create or exacerbate. A second example involves the concern within global health ethics regarding the professional virtues that are considered important for health care providers from high-income countries seeking to work in low-income settings, such as humility and capacity for introspection. While each of these examples offers ethical perspectives to advance global health, they fall outside the scope of dignity-oriented human rights.

Rare examples exist whereby the fields of human rights and global health ethics may stand in conflict with each other. For instance, a dominant value within some global health ethics perspectives is the role of charity (based on the ethical principle of beneficence) as one of the mechanisms through which to respond to global ills (see Chapter 3). However, this orientation of providing support to those in need based on the kindness of the giver and her/his sympathy for the recipient is at odds with a rights-based approach that frames responses in terms of meeting the inalienable human rights of all individuals. This distinction is important because the implications for action resulting from each rationale may be vastly different.

A more productive lens seeks to understand the complementarities of the two fields. First, global health ethics can reinforce the normative claims of international human rights law. While many aspects of human rights law are legally binding, some dimensions are more controversial, less developed, and thus more difficult to enforce. In these instances, ethical arguments can serve to bolster these normative claims and promote their acceptance as law. For example, at present, international human rights law is only weakly applicable to corporate actors. In spite of this, there are growing calls for greater corporate responsibilities regarding human rights in various areas (Forman and Kohler 2012). Such efforts are exemplified in the emergence of global corporate responsibility initiatives, such as the United Nations Global Compact and the International Labour Organization's *Tripartite Declaration of Principles Concerning Multinational Enterprises and Social Policy* (ILO 1978). However, these processes are elucidating 'soft law' principles on human rights with which companies should comply, and have little formal legal status. Similarly, in 2008 the UN Special Rapporteur on the Right to Health released a report entitled *Human Rights Responsibilities for Pharmaceutical Companies in Relation to Access to Medicines* (UNHRC 2008). These duties are not articulated as peremptory duties with which companies "must" comply, but as actions they "should" undertake. The guidelines offer a framework of ethical conduct for the pharmaceutical industry in a range of areas, including access to medicines. While these responsibilities are couched in the language of rights, they are more appropriately classified as ethical as opposed to legal duties. The guidelines offer the pharmaceutical industry greater precision regarding their ethical conduct in a range of areas, and offer social actors a yardstick by which to measure the ethical actions of the industry. The combined effect of these guidelines may be to strengthen both human rights and ethical frameworks in this area, and to contribute towards a public conception of corporate responsibility, which may, in the long run, lead to greater legal enforceability of these duties.

Second, global health ethics can broaden the advocacy framework of human rights. A critical global health ethics seeks to locate phenomena within social, political, economic and historical contexts. In particular, such an approach understands dilemmas as arising from institutional arrangements and power structures (see Chapters 1–3) (Callahan and Jennings 2002). Adding these complementary forms of argumentation to rights-oriented human dignity arguments can result in strengthened advocacy calls for action. For example, the unanimous adoption of the Millennium Development Goals (MDGs) by all UN member states in 2001 reflects states' responsibilities to realize rights through both domestic and international action. MDG 8, "A global partnership for development", calls on high-income countries, in particular, to advance development through various means including improved systems of trade, debt and aid. While human rights obligations provide one justification for wealthy countries to comply, a global health ethics approach can illuminate a broader range of rationales for rich country action in fulfilling MDG 8, such as equity and solidarity, and utilitarian self-interest arguments based on health, security or economic returns. Equally relevant is reasoning from critics such as Benatar et al. (2003) and Pogge (2003), who argue that the past and present policies of wealthy nations have created and maintained poverty and ill health and, therefore, that wealthy nations bear a commensurate responsibility to help alleviate these problems.

Third, global health ethics can assist in resolving the "human rights versus public health" debate. Inherent to this debate is a critique of human rights as being overly individualistic, which, it is argued, can detract from the population-level goals of public health (De Cock et al. 2002). While it is true that rights are individually held entitlements, rights claims also hold strongly collective elements. For example, the individual right to vote cannot be realized without a collective democratic system. Similarly, certain individual claims to the right to health cannot be met without an adequate collective health care system. A concern within public health is the extent to which individual rights can "trump" these collective interests and, conversely, when it is appropriate to limit individual rights in the service of collective health. Different jurisdictions attempt to achieve this balance in different ways: the liberty-oriented model embraced by the US views rights as absolute and able to trump all competing public interests, whereas the approach advanced in international human rights law and other constitutional jurisdictions, such as Canada and South Africa, seeks to balance competing individual rights and collective interests with attention to both human rights principles and the impact of such limitations on individual rights and collective interests.

Since the 1980s, international human rights has articulated the Siracusa Principles, which indicate that rights can be limited in service of public health provided that such limitations are both necessary and proportional, which themselves require ethical justification (UN ECOSOC 1985). A current example of the human rights versus public health debate has occurred in the argument around patient-initiated (opt-in) versus routine (opt-out) HIV testing. This topic has received impassioned attention from both public health and human rights experts (Csete et al. 2004). Public health experts have charged that "human-rights based approaches to HIV/AIDS prevention might have reduced the role of public health and social justice, which offer a more applied and practical framework for HIV/AIDS prevention and care in Africa's devastating epidemic" (DeCock et al. 2002: 67) Ironically, the Siracusa Principles, which are human rights norms, provide weighty support for an opt-out approach to HIV testing, which has traditionally been understood as a predominantly public health position. Nonetheless, human rights advocates have come to realize that in high HIV-prevalence settings, routine testing can be seen as both "necessary" and "proportional" provided that appropriate counselling and protection against adverse outcomes is provided. Thus the Siracusa Principles offer to resolve apparent dichotomies between public health's primary mandate of protecting population health and the human rights imperative to protect individual rights (Gruskin and Loff 2002). These two goals are not necessarily in conflict and, in most cases, are mutually reinforcing. Articulating these principles as ethical norms may strengthen their acceptance and application by those who view human rights as imposing unacceptable obstacles to public health practice.

E) How human rights advances global health ethics

In a reciprocal and reinforcing way, human rights can advance global health ethics. First, human rights emphasize the importance of upstream determinants of health. The 1978 *Declaration of Alma-Ata* described health as "a social goal whose realization requires the action of many social and economic sectors in addition to the health sector" (WHO 1978). From this perspective, the necessary preconditions of health also include those social and environmental components necessary for wellbeing, a view reflected in the 1986 *Ottawa Charter for Health Promotion*, which proposes that "the fundamental conditions and resources for health are peace, shelter, education, food, income, a stable ecosystem, sustainable resources, social justice and equity" (WHO 1986). However, debate continues to flourish regarding the relative significance of the various factors, particularly the importance of "upstream" structural factors such as socio-economic status in comparison with individualistic, behavioural factors such as exercise (Krieger 1994; Szreter 1998; Tesh 1998). This debate is far from theoretical; the answer to the question of *what determines health* has far-reaching implications for governments in terms of policies, expenditures and programming. Furthermore, arguments in favour of individualistic determinants of health shift responsibility and hence cost from the state to individuals.

The field of human rights can bring several decades of debate over the right to health to bear on this public health dialogue on the determinants of health. In particular, human rights can contribute to the public health debate over the relative value of upstream versus downstream (or distal versus proximal) determinants of health by offering a perspective that explicitly encompasses structural, system-level forces. This conception of health as part of a fundamental developmental package is reflected in the UNCESCR's General Comment 14 (2000). Furthermore, the right to health is understood as *indivisible* from other rights. That is, the right to health may be fully achieved only by realizing other human rights. The notion of indivisibility can contribute to the current health policy debate around determinants of health by reinforcing the central role of broader structural factors related to power and oppression in society.

Second, human rights emphasize the obligations of states toward their citizens. At a time when many high-income country governments are reducing public expenditures on health, and after decades of structural adjustment programmes that have forced the same neoliberal reasoning on developing countries, a refocus on states' legal obligations progressively to realize the right to health of all citizens offers added ammunition in both advocating for public health and, where necessary, litigating for specific health services. This is particularly salient for the ongoing debates over what constitutes healthy public policy, including the role of the private sector in delivering health care. That is, global health ethics analyses of public policy for health in both resource-rich and resource-poor countries can be informed by human rights doctrine regarding the ultimate responsibility for health resting with governments, in contrast to the alternative perspectives that view health as a commodity that ought to be regulated by the market. This perspective is reflected in numerous recent global health policy outcomes, including the 2011 *Rio Political Declaration on the Social Determinants of Health* (WHO 2011) and the *UN Political Declaration on the Prevention and Control of Non-Communicable Diseases* (United Nations 2011).

Third, human rights contributes to recognizing the protection of rights as itself a determinant of health. Global health ethics is concerned with identifying and advancing ideas about what ought to be done to improve the health of societies. Mann's thesis about the interconnectedness of health and human rights contributes to the understanding of what makes people healthy or ill (Mann et al. 1999). This recognition that the protection of human rights is itself an important determinant of health is largely absent from the discourse on determinants. However, this has been shown to be a crucial factor in health promotion and disease prevention in contemporary problems like reproductive and sexual health (Freedman 1999). Furthermore, the recognition of human rights as a determinant of health opens up avenues for intervention in the pursuit of improved public health that may not have been realized in the past.

F) Conclusion

Actors within the fields of public health, ethics and human rights can gain analytic tools by embracing the untapped potential for collaboration inherent in such a combined approach. As a relatively mature field, human rights offers the field of global health ethics the benefits of increasingly well-developed notions of state responsibility with respect to health, and an obligatory legal framework for action. Conversely, global health ethics offers human rights a strengthened ethical framework for action, broader justifications for claiming cooperative action in relation to health, and increased acceptance of collective ethical duties towards global public health. We argue that the two approaches in tandem offer a strengthened normative basis for the achievement of global health equity.

In this light, we call for further research to advance understanding and applications of the intersections of human rights and global health ethics, including in relation to: (1) limitations of rights in service of global health interests, (2) responses to new and emerging pandemics, and (3) the legal and ethical basis for articulating the responsibilities of state and non-state actors towards *global* health.

References

African Union (1981) *African Charter on Human and People's Rights, 27 June 1981*. Nairobi: African Union.

Benatar, S.R., Daar, A.S. and Singer, P.A. (2003) 'Global health ethics: the rationale for mutual caring', *International Affairs*, 79(1): 107–38.

Beyrer, C. and Pizer, H.F. (eds) (2007) *Public Health and Human Rights: Evidence-Based Approaches*. Baltimore, MD: Johns Hopkins University Press.

Callahan, D. and Jennings, B. (2002) 'Ethics and public health: forging a strong relationship', *American Journal of Public Health*, 92(2): 169–76.

Consortium for Health and Human Rights (1998) 'A call to action on the 50th anniversary of the Universal Declaration of Human Rights', *Journal of the American Medical Association*, 280(5): 462–64.

Constitutional Court of South Africa (2002) *Minister of Health and Others v Treatment Action Campaign and Others*. Johannesburg: Constitutional Court of South Africa.

Council of Europe (1961) *The European Social Charter, 18 October 1961*. Strasbourg: Council of Europe.

Csete, J., Schleifer, R. and Cohen, J. (2004) '"Opt-out" testing for HIV in Africa: a caution', *Lancet*, 363(9407): 493–94.

DeCock, K.M., Mbori-Ngacha, D. and Marum, E. (2002) 'Shadow on the continent: public health and HIV/AIDS in Africa in the 21st century', *Lancet*, 360(9326): 67–72.

Farmer, P. (2008) 'Challenging orthodoxies: the road ahead for health and human rights', *Health and Human Rights*, 10(1).

Forman, L. (2012) 'A Rights-Based Approach to Global Health Policy: What Contribution can Human Rights Make to Achieving Equity?', in Brown, G., Yarney, G. and Wamala, S. (eds), *The Handbook of Global Health Policy*. West Sussex: Wiley-Blackwell.

Forman, L. (2011) 'Making the case for human rights in global health education, research and policy', *Canadian Journal of Public Health*, 102(3): 207–9.

Forman, L. and Bomze, S. (2012) 'International human rights law and the right to health: an overview of legal standards and accountability mechanisms', in: Blackman, G. et al. (eds), *The Right to Health: Theory and Practice*. Lund: Studentlitteratur AB.

Forman, L. and Kohler, J.C. (eds) (2012) *Access to Medicines as a Human Right: What Implications for the Pharmaceutical Industry?* Toronto: University of Toronto Press.

Freedman, L.P. (1999) 'Censorship and manipulation of family planning information: an issue of human rights and women's health', in: Mann, J., Gruskin, S., Grodin, M.A. and Annas, G.J. (eds), *Health and Human Rights: A Reader*. New York: Routledge.

Gloppen, S. (2008) 'Litigation as a strategy to hold governments accountable for implementing the right to health', *Health and Human Rights*, 10(2): 21–36.

Gruskin, S. and Loff, B. (2002) 'Do human rights have a role in public health work?', *Lancet*, 360(9348): 1880.

Gruskin, S., Mills, E.J. and Tarantola, D. (2007) 'History, principles, and practice of health and human rights', *Lancet*, 370(9585): 449–55.

Harvard School of Public Health (n.d.) 'Health and Human Rights Database', Harvard School of Public Health. www.hsph.harvard.edu/pihhr/resources_hhrdatabase.html

Henkin, L. (1990) *The Age of Rights*. New York: Columbia University Press.

Hogerzeil, H.V. et al. (2006) 'Is access to essential medicines as part of the fulfillment of the right to health enforceable through the courts?', *Lancet*, 368(9532): 305–11.

Hunt, P. (2006) 'The human right to the highest attainable standard of health: new opportunities and challenges', *Transactions of the Royal Society of Tropical Medicine and Hygiene*, 100(7): 603–7.

Hunt, P. and MacNaughton, G. (2006) *Impact Assessments, Poverty and Human Rights: A Case Study Using the Right to the Highest Attainable Standard of Health, Health and Human Rights*, Working Paper Series No. 6. Geneva: World Health Organization and UNESCO.

International Council of Nurses (1998) 'Position statement on nurses and human rights', International Council of Nurses. www.icn.ch/images/stories/documents/publications/position_statements/E10_Nurses_Human_Rights.pdf

ILO (1978) *Tripartite Declaration of Principles Concerning Multinational Enterprises and Social Policy*, November 1977. Geneva: International Labour Organization.

Krieger, N. (1994) 'Epidemiology and the web of causation: has anyone seen the spider?', *Social Science and Medicine*, 39(7): 887–903.

Mann, J., Gruskin, S., Grodin, M.A. and Annas, G.J. (eds) (1999) *Health and Human Rights: A Reader*. New York: Routledge.

Mutua, M.W. (2001) 'J. Shaund Watson – *Theory and Reality in the International Protection of Human Rights* (Book Review)', *American Journal of International Law*, 95(1): 255–56.

Nixon, S. and Forman, L. (2008) 'Exploring the synergies between human rights and public health ethics: a whole greater than the sum of its parts?', *BMC International Health and Human Rights*, 8(2).

OHCHR (2010) 'Special Rapporteur on the right of everyone to the enjoyment of the highest attainable standard of physical and mental health', Office of the United Nations High Commissioner for Human Rights. www.ohchr.org/EN/Issues/Health/Pages/SRRightHealthIndex.aspx

Pogge, T.W. (2003) 'Responsibilities for poverty-related ill health', *Ethics and International Affairs*, 16(2): 71–79.

Risse, T., Ropp, S.C. and Sikkink, K. (eds) (1999) *The Power of Human Rights: International Norms and Domestic Change*. Cambridge: Cambridge University Press.

Rodriguez-Garcia, R. and Akhter, M.N. (2000) 'Human rights: the foundation of public health practice', *American Journal of Public Health*, 90(5): 693–94.

Singh, J.A., Govender, M. and Mills, E.J. (2007) 'Health and human rights 2: do human rights matter to health?', *Lancet*, 370(9586): 521–27.

Statistics South Africa (2010) *Mid Year Population Estimates 2010*. Pretoria: Statistics South Africa.

Szreter, S. (1998) 'The importance of social intervention in Britain's mortality decline', *Society for Social History of Medicine*, 1(1): 1–38.

Tesh, S. (1998) *Hidden Argument: Political Ideology and Disease Prevention Policy*. New Brunswick: Routledge.

UNCESCR (2000) *General Comment No. 14: The Right to the Highest Attainable Standard of Health*, 11 August 2000. New York: United Nations Committee on Economic, Social and Cultural Rights.

UN ECOSOC (1985) *Siracusa Principles on the Limitation and Derogation Provisions in the International Covenant on Civil and Political Rights*. New York: United Nations Economic and Social Council.

UN General Assembly (2007) *Convention on the Rights of Persons with Disabilities*, 24 January 2007. New York: United Nations.

United Nations (1945) 'Preamble', in: *Charter of the United Nations*, 26 June 1945. New York: United Nations.

— (1948) *Universal Declaration of Human Rights*. New York: United Nations.

— (1965) *International Convention on the Elimination of Racial Discrimination*, 21 December 1965. New York: United Nations.

— (1966) *International Covenant on Economic, Social, and Cultural Rights*, 16 December 1966. New York: United Nations.

— (1979) *Convention on the Elimination of All Forms of Discrimination against Women*, 18 December 1979. New York: United Nations.

— (1988) *Additional Protocol to the American Convention on Human Rights in the Area of Economic, Social, and Cultural Rights (Protocol of San Salvador)*. New York: United Nations.

— (1989) *International Convention on the Rights of the Child*, 20 November 1989. New York: United Nations.

— (1993) *Vienna declaration and programme of action*. In: *World Conference on Human Rights*, Vienna, 25 June 1993. New York: United Nations.

— (2011) *Political Declaration of the High-level Meeting of the General Assembly on the Prevention and Control of Non-communicable Diseases*, 16 September 2011. New York: United Nations.

UNHRC (2008) *Human Rights Responsibilities for Pharmaceutical Companies in Relation to Access to Medicines*. Report of the Special Rapporteur on the Right of Everyone to the Enjoyment of Physical and Mental Health. New York: United Nations Human Rights Council.

WHO (1948) 'Preamble', in: *Constitution of the World Health Organization*, 22 July 1946. Geneva: World Health Organization.

— (1978) 'Declaration of Alma-Ata', in: *International Conference on Primary Health Care, 6–12 September 1978*. Geneva: World Health Organization.

— (1986) 'Ottawa Charter for Health Promotion', in: *First International Conference on Health Promotion*, 21 November 1986. Geneva: World Health Organization.

— (2011) *Rio Political Declaration on the Social Determinants of Health*, 21 October 2011. Geneva: World Health Organization.

World Medical Association (1999) *Resolution on the Inclusion of Medical Ethics and Human Rights in the Curriculum of Medical Schools Worldwide*. Ferney-Voltaire: World Medical Association.

Yamin, A.E. and Gloppen, S. (eds) (2011) *Litigating health rights: Can courts bring more justice to health?* Cambridge, MA: Harvard University Press.

5 Global health governance and ethics

Jerome Amir Singh

Objectives

- To provide an introduction to governance for global health practitioners
- To discuss infection control international governance strategies for pandemic management
- To consider the role of civil society in shaping governance

A) Introduction

Governance structures mediate what the various actors can and cannot do within global health. Often academics, students and advocates want to see something changed or something new developed, but are unaware of how things work. This chapter aims to introduce the global health practitioner to governance.

In broad terms, governance can be defined as the actions and means adopted by a society to promote collective action and deliver collective solutions in pursuit of common goals (Dodgson et al. 2002). Governance includes regulation by states (nation states, intergovernmental organizations); regulation by self-organization (private sector and civil society); and hybrid forms of regulation, including cooperation by, and interplay between, states and international organizations, private sector and civil society (Kohlmorgen 2005). Health governance concerns the actions and means adopted by a society to organize itself in the promotion and protection of the health of its population (Dodgson et al. 2002). For a glossary of terms see Table 5.1.

Global health – aimed at improving health for all people (Institute of Medicine 2009) – is concerned with the role and responsibilities of states and interstate bodies, such as the United Nations (UN) and its agencies, international financial institutions such as the World Bank and International Monetary Fund, political groupings like the G-8 and G-20, private foundations, donors and international non-governmental organizations (NGOs). It is evident that the nature and scope of international cooperation has changed dramatically over the past century (see Chapter 1). The

Table 5.1 Glossary of governance terminology

Instrument	Example
Charter/Constitution – a set of foundation principles upon which an organization or body is governed	Charter of the United Nations
Mission statement – comprises a set of fundamental beliefs or guiding principles that defines what an organization is, why it exists, its reason for being	Hospital mission statement
Policy – rules for decision-making and action; not legally enforceable, but usually internally binding within an organization or body	National Department of Health policy on primary health care
Resolution – consensus statement of principles which may or may not be binding	United Nations Security Council Chapter 7 Resolutions (binding) World Health Assembly Resolutions (not binding)
Code – a set of rules (for example, of conduct) promulgated by a body or organization, which is usually binding on members	Professional association code of conduct
Declaration – a set of non-binding guidance points proposed by an organization or body	World Medical Association *Declaration of Helsinki* (2008)
Guideline – a set of non-binding recommendations	WHO guidance documents
Regulations – a set of rules, usually with binding effect	International Health Regulations (2005)
Protocol – a set of regulations or boundaries to operation, recommended by a Convention or Commission, in order to comply with the agreement, convention or treaty; binding on parties who agree to ratify or accede to it	Kyoto Protocol to the United Nations Framework Convention on Climate Change
Treaty – a written agreement between two or more states or Sovereigns, governed by international law	North American Free Trade Agreement
Convention – an agreement that has been drafted by or falling under the auspices of an international, independent organization; binding on parties who ratify or accede to it	Framework Convention on Tobacco Control

recognition by states that they are no longer effective in regulating health independently has necessitated a governance system that encompasses state and non-state actors (Koplan et al. 2009), as well as interstate bodies and international NGOs. "Global health governance" has been defined as "the totality of collective regulations to deal with international and transnational interdependence problems in health" (Hein et al. 2005). It includes the use of formal and informal institutions, rules, and processes by states, intergovernmental organizations and non-state actors to deal with challenges to health that require cross-border collective action (Fidler 2010).

This chapter begins with a brief outline of how global health governance evolved as a discipline. This is followed by an overview of the World Health Organization (WHO) and a review of the role the WHO and other interstate agencies play in global zoonoses governance. This is followed by an overview of infection-control strategies. The chapter concludes with three case studies.

B) Genesis of global health governance

In the mid-nineteenth century, expanding trade and travel between nations saw states initiating dialogue and negotiations on health threats considered to be of international significance, such as plague, cholera and yellow fever. This evolved to collective action on other health threats, such as mitigating pollution in rivers and lakes bordered by two or more countries, protecting the health of combatants during war (now referred to as international humanitarian law), and protecting workers from occupational safety and health risks, an issue now governed by the International Labour Organization. While the WHO is the lead UN agency on global health matters, several players, including other agencies in the UN system (such as the UN International Children's Emergency Fund, UNICEF), have since become major players in the global health arena (Table 5.2).

C) World Health Organization

In the wake of World War II, in 1948 the UN created a specialized health agency, the World Health Organization, to exercise leadership on global health issues. As of 2012, the WHO has 194 member states and is headquartered in Geneva, Switzerland. The World Health Assembly (WHA) is the decision-making body of the WHO and meets annually in Geneva. It is attended by delegates from all WHO Member States and focuses on a specific health agenda prepared by the Executive Board. The WHA's main functions are to determine the policies of the WHO, appoint the WHO Director-General, supervise financial policies, and review and approve the proposed WHO programme budget.

Its constitution requires the WHO to be the "directing and coordinating authority on public health" (Art. 2) and endows the organization with extensive powers (such as the power to pass treaties and regulations), to proactively promote the attainment of "the highest possible level of health." Once adopted by the WHA, the adopted regulations and conventions apply to all WHO member countries, even those that voted against it, unless the government specifically notifies WHO that it rejects the regulation/ convention or accepts it with reservations (Gostin and Mok 2009). Despite being

Table 5.2 Major players in the global health arena (reproduced with permission from Fidler 2010)

Player category	Examples	
States	Great powers	United States, China
	Emerging powers	India, Brazil
	Developed states	Britain, Canada, Germany, Japan, Norway
	Developing countries	Bangladesh, Indonesia, Kenya, Venezuela
	Failing or failed states	Congo, Haiti, Zimbabwe, Somalia
IGOs	Multilateral	ILO, UN, UNAIDS, UNICEF, World Bank, WHO, WTO
	Regional	African Union, ASEAN, European Union
PPPs	Mechanisms to increase access to health technologies	AMCV; GAVI Alliance; Global Fund; IFFIm
	Drug and vaccine development partnerships	Drugs for Neglected Diseases Initiative, International AIDS Vaccine Initiative, Medicines for Malaria Venture, Malaria Vaccine Initiative, TB Alliance
Non-state actors	Philanthropic foundations	Bloomberg Initiative, Carter Center, Clinton Foundation, Gates Foundation, Rockefeller Foundation
	NGOs and civil society groups	Amnesty International, Médecins sans Frontières, Human Rights Watch, Oxfam
	Multinational corporations	Food and beverage, pharmaceutical, and tobacco companies

Abbreviations:
AMCV – Advance Market Commitment for Vaccines
ASEAN – Association of Southeast Asian Nations
GAVI – Global Alliance for Vaccines and Immunisation
IFFIm – International Finance Facility for Immunisation
IGO – international governmental organization
ILO – International Labour Organization
NGO – non-governmental organization
PPP – public–private partnership
TB – tuberculosis
UN – United Nations
UNAIDS – Joint United Nations Programme on HIV/AIDS
UNICEF – United Nations International Children's Emergency Fund
WHO – World Health Organization
WTO – World Trade Organization

equipped with these extensive powers by its constitution, the WHO has been heavily criticized for its reluctance to enact and apply stronger international health governance mechanisms (Lakin 1997; Taylor 2004; Fidler 2005; Gostin and Mok 2009). Since its establishment, the WHA has adopted only three international instruments:

- World Health Regulation No. 1, *Nomenclature with Respect to Diseases and Causes of Death*, which formalized a by-then long-established international process on the classification of disease (WHO 1990). Now known as the *International Classification of Diseases* (ICD), the ICD is *recommendatory* rather than obligatory.
- World Health Regulation No. 2, the International Health Regulations (IHR), dates back to a series of international sanitary conferences held in Europe during the second half of the nineteenth century to address the transboundary effects of infectious diseases. The work initiated by the international sanitary conferences eventually yielded the *International Sanitary Regulations* (ISR), which the WHA adopted in 1951. The ISR applied only to cholera, plague and yellow fever, and were eventually renamed the *International Health Regulations* in 1969. The IHR were extensively revised in 2005 (www.who.int/ihr/en), with a primary focus on "public health emergencies of international concern," defined as "a public health risk to other States through the international spread of disease" (WHO 2005, IHR Art. 1). The IHR is *binding* in nature.
- The *Framework Convention on Tobacco Control* (FCTC) was adopted by the WHO in 2003. The FCTC is aimed at protecting present and future generations from "the devastating health, social, environmental and economic consequences of tobacco consumption and exposure to tobacco smoke" (Art. 3). It adopts multidimensional strategies, including demand reduction, supply reduction and tort litigation (Gostin and Mok 2009). The FCTC is *binding* on ratifying countries.

Because of its poor record in yielding binding governance instruments, the WHO has been criticized as being "highly skewed towards recommendations over treaties and regulations" (Gostin and Mok 2009). Recommendations can take various forms, but two primary types include resolutions and codes of conduct (Gostin and Mok 2009). Non-binding instruments of this nature are referred to as "soft law." Since its founding, the WHO has also assumed a support role to governments through a variety of initiatives, including the publication and dissemination of guidelines and the provision of technical advice.

Pandemic management has emerged as one of the WHO's major concerns in recent years, with the emergence of diseases that can be transmitted between animals and humans (zoonoses diseases), such as severe acute respiratory syndrome (SARS), swine flu and avian flu. It is thus important to briefly consider global zoonoses infection control governance and related containment strategies.

D) Zoonoses infection control governance

The WHO defines zoonoses as diseases and infections that are naturally transmitted between vertebrate animals and humans. Zoonoses management falls under the mandate of three specialized international agencies:

World Health Organization

As noted above, the WHO is the lead UN agency for global human health. The mandate of the IHR (2005) has been expanded beyond cholera, yellow fever and plague (the narrow focus of its previous incarnation), and now applies to zoonoses outbreaks. Some of the containment strategies outlined in the IHR, such as quarantine and isolation, are discussed below.

Food and Agriculture Organization (FAO)

Headquartered in Rome, Italy, the FAO is a specialized agency of the UN that leads international efforts to defeat hunger. However, its mandate also includes zoonoses control, particularly in relation to agricultural animals. In 1994, the FAO established an Emergency Prevention System for Transboundary Animal and Plant Pests and Diseases, focusing on the control of diseases such as rinderpest, foot-and-mouth disease and avian flu. This system is intended to help governments coordinate their responses to transboundary zoonoses threats.

World Organisation for Animal Health (OIE)

Headquartered in Paris, France, the World Organisation for Animal Health [originally *Office International des Epizooties* (International Office of Epizootics) and still known by its historical acronym] is the intergovernmental organization responsible for improving animal health worldwide. Created by an international agreement, the OIE is the sole reference organization for animal health. Its mandate includes setting standards for animal disease surveillance and animal health and welfare, with the objective of providing a scientific basis for safe international trade in animals and animal products and improving animal health and welfare worldwide. The World Trade Organization, under the Agreement on the Application of Sanitary and Phytosanitary Measures, formally recognizes the OIE as the reference organization responsible for establishing international standards relating to animal diseases, including zoonotic diseases.

In response to a rise in zoonoses threats such as H5N1 and H1N1, the WHO, FAO and OIE have published a series of guidelines, independently and in collaboration with each other and other relevant international agencies, to govern zoonoses threats (FAO 2003, 2009; FAO and OIE 2004; OIE and FAO 2007; FAO et al. 2008). Some of these responses include pandemic infection control strategies that impact on human liberties. These containment strategies are reviewed briefly here.

E) Pandemic management: infection control governance strategies

Some of the earliest examples of health regulation came in the form of involuntary isolation, as early societies isolated lepers and others suspected of carrying diseases. While isolation was practiced by early societies, the word "quarantine" has Italian origins, meaning "forty days," the historical period of time a ship or individuals suspected of carrying plague would have to be isolated from those who were known not to carry the disease in the mid-1300s. Surprisingly, despite major advances in diagnostics and prophylaxis since the fourteenth century, isolation and quarantine are still features of modern infection control and are loosely referred to as "social distancing" strategies (Table 5.3).

Table 5.3 Summary of infection control governance strategies (adapted from Singh 2008)

Pandemic management strategy	Definition
Quarantine	The separation and restriction of movement of persons who, while not yet ill, have been exposed to an infectious agent and therefore may become infectious (CDC 2004).
Isolation	The separation of persons who have a specific infectious illness from those who are healthy, and the restriction of the movement of the sick to stop their spread of that illness (CDC 2004).
Voluntary isolation	Occurs when, after appropriate counseling (if necessary), an infected individual voluntarily isolates him/herself from others who are not infected to prevent the infection spreading to the latter. This may take the form of solitary confinement (where the infected individual has no unprotected physical contact with others) or group confinement (where the infected individual shares cohabitation and facilities, and intermingles with others afflicted with the same infection).
Involuntary isolation	Sometimes referred to as 'therapeutic detention'. Applies to infected individuals who refuse to voluntarily isolate themselves to prevent their infection spreading to others. In these instances, the non-cooperative individual may be forcibly confined to a designated setting. Involuntary isolation/enforced hospitalization should be considered only as a last resort.
Incarceration	Although the term is sometimes used in a medical context to refer to isolation (Burman et al. 1997), from a governance perspective it conventionally refers to the imprisonment of individuals who have been tried and convicted of a crime, or to those who violate a court order. This can include non-compliant patients, although their incarceration will raise human rights and public health concerns.

Social distancing has been described as the practice of "increasing the physical space between individuals or infected populations with the aim of delaying spread of disease" (WHO 2006). Social distancing strategies constitute the backbone of public health law in many countries, allowing authorities to act decisively in the face of health threats to the wider public, including those of a trans-boundary nature, even if doing so impinges on an individual's rights. The most common forms of social distancing are isolation, detention, quarantine and incarceration (CDC 2004). While these strategies have in common the confinement of individuals or the restriction of their mobility rights, and are commonly used interchangeably, each is subtly distinct. Unfortunately, the misappropriate use of infection control containment terminology can give rise to concerns amongst human rights activists, who justifiably fear that the criminalization of infection may stigmatize diseases and drive them underground. It is thus important to outline their respective natures.

F) Ethical, human rights and social implications of public health containment strategies

While the above-mentioned containment strategies are arguably effective and have been incorporated into domestic public health governance frameworks, they raise numerous ethical, human rights and social concerns.

Confinement and ethics

Since the early 1970s, the principles of biomedical ethics have been touted as the essential benchmarks of good clinical practice and health research. According to these principles, health practitioners are expected to uphold, amongst others, the patient's right to autonomy (which stresses that mentally competent patients have the right to determine the course of their own health) and non-maleficence (which stresses that patients have the right not to be harmed). However, both principles are violated if authorities forcibly confine non-cooperative infected patients to designated facilities to prevent their infection from spreading to others. Such an outcome is untenable as it will mean that while a containment measure may be legal, it would be unethical according to the biomedical ethics paradigm. Accordingly, the past decade has seen the emergence of various proposed principles of "public health ethics."

Public health ethics is increasingly being seen as a distinct branch of bioethics and has been described as

> [t]he principles and values that help guide actions among public health system actors, which are designed to promote health and prevent injury and disease in the population. The principal values of public health ethics include the salience of population health, safety, and welfare; fairness and equity in the distribution of services; and respect for the human rights of individuals and groups.
>
> (Gostin 2003)

Nancy Kass (2001), James Childress (Childress et al. 2002), Ross Upshur (2002) and Lawrence Gostin (2003), amongst others, have proposed various frameworks of public health ethics – analytical tools of sorts akin to the four principles of biomedical ethics – designed to help public health professionals consider the specific ethical implications of proposed public health interventions, policy proposals, research projects and health programmes. The following seven-step framework is a brief attempt to synthesize their respective proposals (Singh 2007):

- What are the public health goals of the proposed project? – the principle of harm prevention and necessity
- How effective is the project known to be in achieving its stated goals? – the principle of effectiveness
- What are the known or potential burdens of the project? – the principle of burden identification
- Can the burdens be minimized? Are there alternative approaches? – the principle of least infringement/restriction/coercion
- Is the project implemented fairly? – the principle of proportionality
- Can the benefits and burdens of the project be fairly balanced? – the principle of public justification and transparency
- Individuals who are affected by public health initiatives should be adequately supported or fairly compensated – the principle of reciprocity

Confinement and human rights

Human rights refers to a set of principles and norms internationally agreed upon by governments that are contained in treaties, conventions, declarations, resolutions, guidelines and recommendations at the international and regional levels. Modern human rights instruments have their source in the 1948 Universal Declaration of Human Rights (see Chapter 4). Although this instrument is not legally binding on countries, it carries considerable moral authority. At first sight, infection control containment strategies appear potentially to violate several rights in this instrument, including Article 3 (Everyone has the right to life, liberty, and security of person); Article 5 (No one shall be subjected to torture or to cruel, inhuman or degrading treatment or punishment); Article 9 (No one shall be subjected to arbitrary arrest, detention or exile); Article 12 (No one shall be subjected to arbitrary interference with his privacy, family, home…); and Article 25 (Everyone has the right to a standard of living adequate for the health and well-being of himself and his family, including …medical care and the necessary social services, and the right to security in the event of… sickness).

However, human rights doctrine also recognizes the limitation of many rights in a public health emergency, provided the measures employed are legitimate, non-arbitrary, publicly rendered and necessary. In this regard, section 25 of the Siracusa Principles on the Limitation and Derogation of Provisions in the International Covenant on Civil and Political Rights holds: "Public health may be invoked as a ground for limiting certain rights in order to allow a state to take measures dealing with a serious threat to the health of the population or individual members of the population. These measures must be aimed specifically at preventing disease or injury or providing care for the sick and injured." A particular issue from a human rights perspective is whether the containment strategy in question represents the least restrictive means to achieve effective infection control and the extent of the belief in the severity of the threat. The restrictions imposed by authorities should also be of limited duration and subject to review.

While the curtailment of rights on the grounds of public health is endorsed by human rights instruments, health workers should also be cognizant of the social implications of such measures.

G) Confinement and social factors

As noted above, public health authorities usually focus primarily on the public health aspects of infection control and rely on judicial and law enforcement authorities for assistance in this regard. However, social factors often lead to individuals resisting confinement measures, and addressing their concerns meaningfully will often hold the key to effective infection control.

For example, in the case of drug-resistant tuberculosis (TB), health authorities may deem the isolation of the infected individual to be the most effective containment strategy. However, that individual may be the primary or sole bread-winner of his/her family, and confinement in a health facility for up to twenty-four months (in the case of multi-drug-resistant, MDR-TB) or indefinitely (in the case of extremely drug-resistant, XDR-TB) will effectively mean that the family of that individual will be deprived of his/her means of livelihood during this period. Similar factors would apply to infected single heads of households with dependants: a prolonged or indefinite confinement in a health facility would likely mean that such dependants would be deprived of their care-giver during that period.

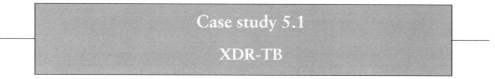

Case study 5.1

XDR-TB

An arriving traveller presents at an international airport with cough and a high fever. Emigration officers realize the individual is a highly infectious defaulting XDR-TB patient who has been placed on an international watch-list. How should the authorities proceed in the matter?

The IHR requires signatory nations to notify WHO of (1) any event that may constitute a public health emergency of international concern (PHEIC); or (2) any significant evidence of public health risks outside their territory that may lead to or cause the international spread of disease (IHR 2005, Art. 6–8). The IHR also requires nations to expand their national health surveillance capacities and implement certain measures for regulating international traffic at airports and other entry points (IHR 2005, Art. 5).

Whether the IHR can or should be used to control TB globally is unresolved because it is not clear whether cases of TB, MDR-TB or XDR-TB constitute a PHEIC (Calian and Fidler 2007). WHO's Global Task Force on XDR-TB has suggested that XDR-TB should not be considered a PHEIC because its origins are attributed to internal state policies and it is not as much of an acute threat as other diseases such as SARS (WHO Global XDR-TB Task Force 2007). However, this position has been challenged (Wilson et al. 2007). There is, however, precedent for considering MDR and XDR-TB as potential PHEICs. In 2007 the USA notified WHO of one person with drug-resistant TB who travelled internationally by commercial aircraft in 2007 as a potential PHEIC (WHO 2007).

Case study 5.2

Cholera outbreak in Zimbabwe

Due to crumbling infrastructure, sewage plants in Zimbabwe begin leaking raw sewage into rivers. Within weeks, thousands of people who rely on the rivers contract cholera. The Zimbabwean government denies that the country is experiencing a cholera pandemic, despite thousands of deaths and sick refugees presenting in bordering countries, and refuses to act on the emergency. Can the international community legally intervene in instances when a state is unwilling or unable to control an epidemic?

The above scenario mirrors what occurred in Zimbabwe in 2008, and raises the question of what recourse populations have in the event of a disaster if their host state is incapable or unwilling to provide basic aid and is reluctant to request international assistance. Currently there is no general convention that governs all aspects of disaster relief, in stark contrast to international humanitarian law, which protects civilians during armed conflicts (Davies 2010). On the question of humanitarian access, international law tends to favour the protection of sovereignty and territorial integrity over the protection of populations (United Nations 2007). However, while international law does not currently govern humanitarian disasters, the WHO's revised IHR (2005) lists cholera as one of the diseases about which states are required to notify WHO, due to its potential serious public health impact and its ability to spread internationally. The IHR requires that states request international assistance if they have insufficient antidotes, drugs, vaccine, protection equipment and financial, human and material resources to contain the disease.

The breakdown of the public health system in Zimbabwe, the case fatality rate of cholera victims, and the speed at which the disease spread in 2008 all pointed to the state being unable to effectively contain the disease outbreak (Davies 2010). In terms of the IHR 2005, Zimbabwe's 2008 cholera outbreak constituted an emergency and the Zimbabwean government had a duty to accept the assistance offered by WHO and various NGOs. In instances where a state still refuses to accept international intervention in the face of a major disease outbreak, the UN Security Council could become involved. The UN High-level Panel on Threats, Challenges, and Change (United Nations 2004) noted that in certain instances:

> [T]he Security Council should be prepared to support the work of WHO investigators or to deploy experts reporting directly to the Council, and if existing International Health Regulations do not provide adequate access for WHO investigations and response coordination, the Security Council should be prepared to mandate greater compliance. In the event that a State is unable to adequately quarantine large numbers of potential carriers, the Security Council should be prepared to support international action to assist in cordon operations. The Security Council should consult with the WHO Director-General to establish the necessary procedures for working together in the event.

Due to the possibility of being classified as a failed state (which would have opened the door to possible UN Security Council intervention), the Zimbabwe government eventually declared the cholera outbreak a national emergency in December 2008, and invited WHO to coordinate a Health Cluster response effort with the cooperation of the Zimbabwe health ministry and other non-governmental agencies.

Case study 5.3

Creating novel strains of H5N1

Scientists create novel, highly transmissible forms of H5N1 and want to publish their methodology and findings. The US government believes publishing the data could constitute a bioterrorism threat and pressurizes the receiving journal to publish a redacted version of the manuscript that does not contain information the government deems sensitive. The scientists and journal object to this proposal. The US government turns to the WHO to intervene in the matter. What governance instruments govern the matter?

As any unintended release of modified H5N1 viruses from laboratories conducting such research would have the potential for serious global consequences, the IHR (2005) could be invoked to prevent and control a possible international spread of H5N1. The application of IHR (2005) to the given scenario would necessitate the countries hosting such research to report the research to the international community, amongst other reporting obligations. Given the potential implications of such reporting, it is essential that the storage and research involving such materials meet appropriate requirements for biosafety and biosecurity. In this regard, aside from IHR (2005), a range of internationally recognized (but non-binding) standards and guidance can be applied by national authorities to assist in defining the appropriate conditions for further work on modified and potentially deadly pathogens:

- WHO (2004) *Laboratory Biosafety Manual*, 3rd edn.
- WHO (2006) *Biorisk Management: Laboratory Biosecurity Guidance*.
- WHO (2010) *Responsible Life Sciences Research for Global Health Security*.
- CEN CWA 15793 (2011) *Laboratory Biorisk Management*.
- CEN CWA 16393 (2011) *Laboratory Biorisk Management – Guidelines for the Implementation of CWA 15793 (2008)*.

Currently, no binding international instrument governs the study of potentially dual-use biological samples and the dissemination of the results thereof. This speaks to a major gap in biosafety and biorisk governance, global health research governance, and public health governance.

H) Conclusion

Global health emphasizes the need for governance that incorporates participation by a broadly defined "global" constituency, and engaging them in collective action through agreed institutions and rules (Dodgson et al. 2002). The global nature of the threat posed by new and re-emerging infectious diseases will require international cooperation between state and non-state actors in identifying, controlling and preventing these diseases. Civil society – often as part of social movements – plays a role in shaping governance, typically through challenging the (in)action of nation states. The task of defining more clearly the potential role of non-state actors within a system of global health governance is challenging, especially as relationships, patterns of influence, and agreed roles among state and non-state actors within an emerging system of global health governance are still emerging. Global health governance will continue to evolve, as stakeholders expand their resources, knowledge and influence.

References

Burman, W.J., Cohn, D.L., Rietmeijer, C.A., Judson, F.N., Sbarbaro, J.A. and Reves, R.R. (1997) 'Short-term incarceration for the management of noncompliance with tuberculosis treatment', *Chest*, 112(1): 57–62.

Calian, P. and Fidler, D.P. (2007) 'The New International Health Regulations and Human Rights', *Global Health Governance*, 1(1).

CDC (2004) *Isolation and Quarantine Fact Sheet*. Atlanta, GA: US Centers for Disease Control. www.cdc.gov/quarantine/quarantineisolation.html

Childress, J.F., Faden, R.R., Gaare, R.D., Gostin, L.O., Kahn, J., Bonnie, R.J., Kass, N.E., Mastroianni, A.C., Moreno, J.D. and Nieburg, P. (2002) 'Public health ethics: mapping the terrain', *Journal of Law, Medicine and Ethics*, 30: 170–78.

Davies, S. (2010) 'Is there an international duty to protect persons in the event of an epidemic?', *Global Health Governance*, 3(2). www.ghgj.org/Davies_Is%20There%20 an%20International%20Duty%20to%20Protect.pdf

Dodgson, R., Lee, K. and Drager, N. (2002) *Global Health Governance: A Conceptual Review*. Geneva: World Health Organization and London School of Hygiene and Tropical Medicine. http://whqlibdoc.who.int/publications/2002/a85727_eng.pdf

FAO (2003) *Veterinary Public Health and Control of Zoonoses in Developing Countries*. www.fao.org/docrep/006/y4962t/y4962t00.htm#Contents

— (2009) *Guidelines for Surveillance of Pandemic H1N1/2009 and other Influenza Viruses in Swine Populations*. www.fao.org/AG/AGAInfo/programmes/en/empres/AH1N1/docs/ h1n1_guidelines_fao.pdf

FAO and OIE (2004) *The Global Framework for the Progressive Control of Transboundary Animal Diseases (GF-TADs)*. www.oie.int/fileadmin/Home/eng/About_us/docs/pdf/GF-TADs_approved_version24May2004.pdf

FAO, OIE, WHO, UN System Influenza Coordination, UNICEF and World Bank (2008) *Contributing to One World, One Health. A Strategic Framework for Reducing Risks of Infectious Diseases at the Animal–Human–Ecosystems Interface*. ftp://ftp.fao.org/ docrep/fao/011/aj137e/aj137e00.pdf

Fidler, D.P. (2005) 'From international sanitary conventions to global health security: the new international health regulations', *Chinese Journal of International Law*, 4(2): 325–92.

— (2010) *The Challenges of Global Health Governance*. Council on Foreign Relations working paper. http://ec.europa.eu/health/eu_world/docs/ev_20111111_rd01_en.pdf

Gostin, L.O. (2003) 'Public health ethics: traditions, profession, and values', *Acta Bioethica*, 9(2): 177–88.

Gostin, L.O. and Mok, E.A. (2009) 'Global health governance report', in: Institute of Medicine Committee on the US Commitment to Global Health, *The US Commitment to Global Health: Recommendations for the Public and Private Sectors*. Washington, DC: National Academies Press, 205–248. www.ncbi.nlm.nih.gov/books/NBK23801/pdf/TOC.pdf

Hein, W., Bartsch, S. and Kohlmorgen, L. (2005) *Global Health Governance: Institutional Changes in the Poverty-oriented Fight of Diseases. A Short Introduction to a Research Project*. www.temple.edu/lawschool/phrhcs/salzburg/Salzburg_GHG.pdf

Institute of Medicine (2009) *The U.S. Commitment to Global Health: Recommendations for the Public and Private Sectors*. Institute of Medicine Committee on the US Commitment to Global Health. www.ncbi.nlm.nih.gov/books/NBK23801/pdf/TOC.pdf

Kass, N.E. (2001) 'An ethics framework for public health', *American Journal of Public Health*, 91(11): 1776–82. doi: 10.2105/AJPH.91.11.1776

Kohlmorgen, L. (2005) *International Organisations and Global Health Governance. The Role of the World Health Organization, World Bank, and UNAIDS*. Working paper presented at the Salzburg Seminar on the Governance of Health, 12/05–12/08/2005. www.temple.edu/lawschool/phrhcs/salzburg/kohlmorgen_salzburg.pdf

Koplan, J.P., Bond, T.C., Merson, M.H., Reddy, K.S., Rodriguez, M.H. et al. (2009) 'Towards a common definition of global health', *Lancet*, 373: 1993–95.

Lakin, A. (1997) 'The legal powers of the World Health Organization', *Medical Law International*, 3(1): 23–49.

OIE and FAO (2007) *Ensuring Good Governance to Address Emerging and Re-emerging Animal Disease Threats*. www.oie.int/fileadmin/Home/eng/Support_to_OIE_Members/docs/pdf/Good_vet_governance.pdf

Singh, J.A. (2007) 'Epidemiology: ethics, advocacy and human rights', in: Joubert, G. and Ehrlich, R.I. (eds), *Epidemiology: A Research Manual for South Africa*. Cape Town: Oxford University Press, 30–38.

— (2008) 'Humanitarian work and infection control: legal, ethical, human rights, and social considerations', in: Biquet, J.-M. (ed.), *Humanitarian Stakes No. 1: MSF Switzerland's Review on Humanitarian Stakes and Practices*. Geneva: Médecins Sans Frontières, 12–22.

Taylor, A. (2004) 'Governing the globalization of public health', *Journal of Law, Medicine & Ethics*, 32(3): 500–8.

United Nations (2004) *A More Secure World: Our Shared Responsibility*. Report of the Secretary-General's High-level Panel on Threats, Challenges and Change, December 2. Fifty-Ninth Session A/59/565, para. 144.

— (2007) *Protection of Persons in the Event of Disasters*, Memorandum by the Secretariat, December 11. General Assembly Sixtieth Session, A/CN.4/590.

Upshur, R. (2002) 'Principles for the justification of public health intervention', *Canadian Journal of Public Health*, 93: 101–3.

WHO (1990) *History of the Development of the ICD (International Classification of Diseases)*. Geneva: World Health Organization. www.who.int/classifications/icd/en/HistoryOfICD.pdf

— (2003) *Framework Convention on Tobacco Control*. Doc. A56/VR/4. Geneva: World Health Organization. http://whqlibdoc.who.int/publications/2003/9241591013.pdf

— (2005) *Revision of the International Health Regulations 2005*. Fifty-Eighth World Health Assembly. Geneva: World Health Organization. www.who.int/csr/ihr/IHRWHA58_3-en.pdf

— (2006) *Programme on Disease Control in Humanitarian Emergencies Communicable Diseases Cluster. Pandemic influenza preparedness and mitigation in refugee and displaced populations. WHO guidelines for humanitarian agencies*. Geneva: World Health Organization. www.who.int/diseasecontrol_emergencies/training/PI_contents_introduction_jan07.pdf

— (2007) 'Extensively drug-resistant tuberculosis (XDR-TB) in United States of America air passenger'. News release, May 30. Geneva: World Health Organization. www.who.int/csr/don/2007_05_30a/en/index.html

WHO Global XDR-TB Task Force (2007) *Control of XDR-TB. Update on progress since the Global XDR-TB Task Force Meeting, 9–10 October 2006*. Geneva: World Health Organization. www.stoptb.org/events/world_tb_day/2007/assets/documents/globaltaskforce_update_feb07.pdf

Wilson, K., Gardam, K., McDougall, C., Attaran, A. and Upshur, R. (2007) 'WHO's response to global public health threats: XDR-TB'. *PLoS Medicine*, 4(7): e246. doi: 10.1371/journal.pmed.0040246; www.plosmedicine.org/article/info:doi/10.1371/journal.pmed.0040246

6 Indigenous health and ethics: lessons for global health

Andrew D. Pinto and Janet Smylie

Objectives

- To understand the health – and determinants of health – of Indigenous peoples globally
- To examine the historic and contemporary impact of colonization on the health of Indigenous peoples
- To introduce select Indigenous concepts relevant to ethics and global health
- To apply lessons learned from the ethics of working with Indigenous peoples to other areas of global health

> We have survived Canada's assault on our identity and our rights... Our survival is a testament to our determination and will to survive as a people. We are prepared to participate in Canada's future – but only on the terms that we believe to be our rightful heritage.
>
> –Wallace Labillois, Council of Elders, Kingsclear, New Brunswick (Royal Commission on Aboriginal Peoples 1996)

A) Introduction

There are over 370 million Indigenous peoples living in over 90 countries around the world (United Nations 2009). The enormous diversity in language, beliefs and cultural practices seen across 5000 distinct communities belies the use of a single term to label them all. Yet these communities share a common history of colonization and marginalization, as well as of resistance against dominant sectors of society. Resistance has occurred particularly through a focus on the preservation of their distinct identities and cultural, economic and political ways of life (UN Permanent Forum on Indigenous Issues n.d.).

While no universal definition of Indigenous peoples has been accepted (WHO 2007a), it is crucial to be mindful of terminology. Being able to define one's community on one's own terms is a central part of self-determination. It preserves the right and power of communities to decide who belongs to them, rather than have this dictated by outsiders (International Work Group for Indigenous Affairs n.d.). Self-identification happens through language that a community has chosen, or through terms it has reclaimed. While it is beyond this chapter to explore the history of terms used and misused to describe Indigenous peoples (Bartlett et al. 2007), Table 6.1 lists some examples. Most definitions will include reference to the relationships of Indigenous peoples to a collective kin group and a current or historic land base. For example, one definition from the Indigenous Physicians Association of Canada is:

> communities, peoples and nations…which, having a historical continuity with pre-invasion and pre-colonial societies that developed on their territories, consider themselves distinct from other sectors of the societies now prevailing on those territories, or part of them. They form, at present, non-dominant sectors of society and are determined to preserve, develop and transmit to future generations their ancestral territories, and their ethnic identity, as a basis of their continued existence as peoples, in accordance with their own cultural patterns, social institutions and legal system.
>
> (Indigenous Physicians Association of Canada and Association of Faculties of Medicine of Canada 2008: 6)

Table 6.1 Terms used when referring to Indigenous peoples in select countries

Country	Terms
Australia	Australian Aborigines
	Aboriginal Australians
	Torres Strait Islanders
	Natives
	Indigenous Australians
Canada	Aboriginal people
	First Nations
	Indians, Status Indians and Non-Status Indians
	Inuit
	Métis
New Zealand	Māori
	Tangata Whenua ('people of the land')
USA	Native Americans
	Tribes
	Indian, American Indians
	Native Hawaiians
	Native Alaskans

In this chapter, we examine the health of Indigenous peoples, intentionally focusing on communities in four high-income settler colonial states: Australia, Canada, New Zealand and the United States (Anderson et al. 2006). We explore the determinants of health of these communities, particularly colonization as a key historic and contemporary determinant. We end by reviewing the emerging body of literature on the ethics of research involving Indigenous communities and discuss how it can be applied to other global health work.

B) The health of Indigenous people globally

The health of Indigenous peoples living in high-income countries has traditionally been considered outside the remit of global health, related in part to the outward-focused gaze of the field (see Chapter 1). However, a growing awareness of the similarities in health issues faced by Indigenous communities in high-income countries and large segments of populations in low-income countries has led to a convergence in theory and practice (University of Victoria Center for Aboriginal Health Research 2010).

As with many marginalized communities, obtaining accurate data on Indigenous peoples is difficult. In many regions of the world they are unrecognized, uncounted and invisible (Stephens et al. 2005; WHO 2007b). Few data are available from some of the countries and regions with the largest numbers of Indigenous peoples, including China, India and Russia. This is related to historical and ongoing efforts by the state to undermine sovereignty and self-determination. Such structural forces are compounded by geographic isolation, often a product of explicit efforts by the dominant community. In addition, definitions of who is Indigenous and who is not are contested, and the large majority of health information systems do not have inclusive and appropriate ways of identifying Indigenous identity. For example, in Canada, assessing the health of Indigenous individuals and communities is hampered by undercounting, exclusion, or a lack of appropriate identifiers on the national census, vital registration data, major health surveys, health service utilization data and data from surveillance systems (Smylie and Anderson 2006; Smylie et al. 2006).

Perhaps the most important set of issues for Indigenous health and social data and data systems is the fact that Indigenous concepts of health and Indigenous peoples are far too often marginalized in the production, analysis, sharing and application of Indigenous data (Smylie et al. 2006). Indigenous peoples have diverse and rich understandings of health that are highly relevant to the current global debates regarding the need to refocus health care systems away from acute care, high-cost treatments towards upstream prevention. For example, in Cree, achieving a state of health and wellbeing might be expressed using the term *mino-pimatisiwin*. This term can be loosely translated into English as "living well". Cree scholar Herman Michell further describes the concept of health and wellbeing as "more than just the absence of disease and the physical, it is about an entire philosophy of life, a way of being, a way of knowing, and way of becoming whole and complete as we move through the different stages of life" (Michell 2005).

Where available, the data indicate that Indigenous communities have worse health and lower social status compared with dominant, non-Indigenous populations

(Montenegro and Stephens 2006; Ohenjo et al. 2006). In a study looking at the health of Indigenous children in Canada, Australia, New Zealand and the United States, a number of disparities consistently appear. Infant mortality rates are 1.7 to four times higher than for non-Indigenous infants. There are much higher rates of sudden infant death syndrome, injuries, accidental death and suicide (Fantus et al. 2009). Infectious diseases are significantly higher, including inner ear infections and respiratory tract infections, and there are higher rates of exposure to environmental contaminants including tobacco smoke (Smylie and Adomako 2009).

Likewise, adults fare worse than their non-Indigenous counterparts. Indigenous peoples are more likely to experience disability, reduced quality of life and death at a younger age (United Nations 2009). In Canada, a gap in life expectancy of approximately seven years exists between Indigenous peoples and the general population, while in New Zealand it is 11 years and in Australia 20 years (United Nations 2009). In Canada, the smoking rate in First Nation adults is more than double the rate in the general Canadian population. The proportion reporting weekly heavy drinking is double, and there are much higher rates of obesity, diabetes and other chronic diseases (Health Canada 2005). Infectious diseases also occur at high rates. For example, the rate of tuberculosis in Indigenous communities in Canada is 35 to 150 times higher than the general population, which is similarly noted among the Sami of Greenland and the Maori of New Zealand (United Nations 2009). HIV and other sexually transmitted diseases occur at disproportionately high rates, particularly among women (Health Canada 2010).

Such health inequities are not unexpected when one looks at their broader determinants. Indigenous peoples' access to health care service is often constrained by financial, geographical and cultural barriers. When services are available, health care staff are often insensitive, discriminatory and unfriendly (Stephens et al. 2006). Across multiple settings, Indigenous individuals have lower incomes, lower educational attainment and higher rates of unemployment (Smylie and Adomako 2009). Finally, the physical environment in which Indigenous peoples live, work and play is often contaminated by pesticides, industrial waste and the residue of extractive industries (United Nations 2009).

Focusing on single factors in isolation does not fully capture how multiple determinants intersect and reinforce one another (WHO 2007b), and may not reflect the holism apparent in Indigenous conceptualizations of health (Nettleton et al. 2007). High levels of poverty, low levels of educational attainment and high rates of unemployment are all causally linked. These, in turn, are determined by access to physical, economic and social resources, political power at the individual and community level, and the actions of external forces such as state governments. All this is shaped by whether Indigenous peoples have realized certain human rights (see Chapter 4) related to self-determination, autonomy and self-government, freedom from discrimination and persecution, and control over education, environment, economic conditions and the land. While these are all enshrined within the United Nations Declaration on the Rights of Indigenous Peoples and other international treaties, they are far from being realized (United Nations 2007). To understand why, we now examine colonialism, which has been implicated at the heart of the current reality of Indigenous peoples (Stephens et al. 2006).

C) Colonization and resistance

Global health scholars will be familiar with the legacy of colonialism as a force that has shaped the health of communities within low-income countries and that continues to be part of the relationship between the North and South (see Chapters 1 and 10). While national liberation from colonial powers occurred in many of these countries beginning in the 1960s, in many ways "Indigenous peoples represent the unfinished business of decolonization" (Wilmer 1993: 197). Despite the denial by some of a history of colonialism (Ljunggren 2009), it is essential to see this as a process that is ongoing and not an isolated part of the historical record.

The impact of colonization in high-income countries has been succinctly described as "resource exploitation of Indigenous lands, residential school syndrome, racism, expropriation of lands, extinguishment of rights, wardship, and welfare dependency" (Alfred 2009: 43). The invasion of traditional lands by European settlers led to a decimation of populations as a result of dispossession and dislocation from traditional lands, social change that included cultural suppression and assimilation, political marginalization and the introduction of new diseases (Anderson et al. 2006).

Colonialism attacked Indigenous societies at all levels. First, communities were removed from the land and their traditional way of life (Cunningham and Stanley 2003). In many cases, this was through direct violence, while in others it was the outcome of treaty negotiations. Treaties were often negotiated under duress and in a manner that resulted in significantly different understandings of what was intended or achieved. The reserve system was born out of these interactions, created as supposed places of protection but following an ideology of "separate development." Importantly, Indigenous peoples typically had no ownership of the land and very few rights if they left the reserve.

Second, cultural systems and practices were criminalized and undermined (Reid 2006). Knowledge about infant, child and family health was typically part of oral histories that were shared verbally and experientially. Overt suppression of Indigenous cultures and languages had an enormous negative impact on this intergenerational transmission of knowledge teaching (Smylie and Adomako 2009). In Canada, legislation mandated the removal of Indigenous children from their homes and their placement in residential schools. Over 150,000 children were placed in such institutions and the mortality rate was approximately 40 per cent. Those who survived were subject to severe forms of abuse, neglect and the active suppression of traditional languages and culture. The removal of children into residential schools was an extreme manifestation of cultural suppression. As noted by a Royal Commission, "The bonds between many hundreds of Aboriginal children and their families and nations were bent and broken, with disastrous results" (Royal Commission on Aboriginal Peoples 1996). Unfortunately, in part due to the traumatic legacy of residential schools, Indigenous children in Canada continue to be removed from homes at very high rates and placed into protective services (Harris et al. 2007).

A third aspect of colonization was fostering dependency "in physical, psychological and financial terms, on the very people and institutions that have caused the near erasure of our existence and who have come to dominate us" (Alfred 2009: 42).

Political and social institutions, such as band or tribal councils, are often funded by state governments and must operate within their constraints. Any movement to change the status quo can be neutralized through defunding. Similarly to many low-income countries where global health activities take place, Indigenous organizations are often kept busy fulfilling the needs of funders – through providing reports, attending meetings and demonstrating change on performance indicators developed externally. The large proportion of Indigenous peoples – both on and off reserve – who are dependent on state welfare undermines self-sufficiency. Simultaneously, significant barriers exist to accessing resources (education, employment) that would enable Indigenous peoples to participate in and control their own lives.

Finally, colonialism as a process of both physical and psychological displacement results in the internalization of oppression, resulting in trauma and self-hatred. Indigenous peoples "bear their past within them" (Said 1993: 212) and "perceive a need to decolonize our minds" (Smith 1999: 23). Internalizing the superior/inferior dichotomy of colonial/Indigenous knowledge, language and cultural practices is perhaps the most devastating aspect of colonialism. It inhibits the reconstitution of the ability to survive and care for individuals and communities, reinforcing a sense that one's community is worthless (Alfred 2009).

Highlighting resistance and resilience is as important a task as documenting the negative impact of colonization. While primary resistance continues against dominant society hegemony over land and resources, Indigenous peoples are also engaged in ideological resistance and the reconstitution of community (Said 1993). This occurs in part through exerting the right to self-determination, through naming and claiming rights, through the restoration of cultural heritage and through opposing racism and discrimination (WHO 2007b). A full account is beyond the scope of this chapter, but resistance occurs through establishing sovereignty (e.g. the Canadian territory Nunavut), winning land claims (e.g. British Columbia, Canada), and preserving language and cultural heritage (e.g. New Zealand language nests). At a local level, resistance manifests in communities that support one another in the face of poverty and discrimination (Silver 2007) and familial disruption (Baskin 2007). Community-led health promotion campaigns to increase smoking cessation (Cancer Care Ontario 2008) and reduce the incidence of diabetes (Potvin et al. 2003) are further examples of how Indigenous peoples are taking back control of their health and wellbeing.

D) "Decolonizing methodologies"

A crucial aspect of resistance by Indigenous peoples has also been reclaiming the ability to define and understand their own communities. Research is a site of this struggle as it is intimately related to protecting and preserving traditional knowledge (Maina 2003). It is also part of the deeper issue of reframing who is able to *know* Indigenous peoples (Said 1979). It should be noted that "aboriginal knowledge has always been informed by research, the purposeful gathering of information and the thoughtful distillation of meaning" (Castellano 2004: 98). As Smith, a Maori scholar, has noted, "Decolonization, however, does not mean and has not meant a total rejection of all theory or research or

Western knowledge. Rather, it is about centring our concerns and our world views and then coming to know and understand theory and research from our own perspectives and for own purposes" (Smith 1999: 39).

Indigenous knowledge that is developed through decolonized methodologies is a powerful alternative, for both colonizer and colonized. "By animating the voices and experiences of the cognitive 'other' and integrating them into the educational process, [Indigenous knowledge] creates a new, balanced centre and a fresh vantage point from which to analyze Eurocentric education and its pedagogies" (Battiste 2005).

Examples of decolonizing methodologies include a community resisting the imposition of an externally developed measure of wellbeing and developing a unique and relevant indicator themselves (Ten Fingers 2005). Another example is the use of life-course epidemiology to integrate biological and social risk processes and to conceptualize how socio-economic determinants of health influence the development of chronic diseases (Estey et al. 2007). A recent example is community-based participatory research that assesses the health of urban Aboriginals using respondent-driven sampling (Smylie et al. 2011).

Decolonizing methodologies is also about respecting and upholding differences in worldviews. Indigenous worldviews place special significance on the idea of the unification of humans with the natural world, and hence displacement from the land is particularly traumatic (Matthews 1997). These worldviews are often centered on the importance of intergenerational relationships, community wellbeing and a holistic understanding of health (Estey et al. 2007). They differ from mainstream Western views of health by focusing not just on the individual, but on the community, the environment (Stephens et al. 2005) and communal health (United Nations 2009). This is part of the reason why considering and addressing the social determinants is so essential.

A review of case studies from around the world that discuss ways to address these social determinants found that successful solutions are holistic – they address spiritual, physical, mental, emotional, cultural, economic, social and environmental factors, and address the individual and the context together (WHO 2007b). The case studies also illustrated the importance of capacity building (Smylie et al. 2006) better data and supporting community resilience. Research projects should lead to increases in real financial support for health and social services and emphasize communal ownership, building strong links with local community networks.

E) Ethical principles from research involving Indigenous communities

Global health practitioners working with marginalized individuals and communities may learn a great deal from Indigenous peoples and the work done on the ethics of research involving Indigenous communities. Given the historical and contemporary relationships between dominant societies and Indigenous peoples, it is not surprising that such ethical guidelines have emerged from grave concerns about the behavior of researchers (Schnarch 2004). Academics have played a central role in establishing the superiority of Western knowledge, of furthering ecological imperialism and cultural appropriation (Ten Fingers 2005). As Smith has stated, "'Research' is probably one of the dirtiest words in the Indigenous world's vocabulary" (Smith 1999: 1). As in many areas within global health (see Chapters 8 and 10), studies have been conducted in Indigenous communities without obtaining community consent. Many examples exist where researchers have published results without first discussing the implications for communities. The approaches used have not always reflected Indigenous worldviews, and have often undermined them as "primitive" or "superstitious". Typically, communities have not benefited from the research that has been conducted upon them. Most concerning, perhaps, have been studies where scientists have collected biological material (e.g. blood, tissue) from Indigenous peoples and analyzed these samples without their explicit permission, sometimes putting forth hypotheses that violate the community's ideas about creation and their connection to the land. Communities have often had to fight for the return of these samples (Dodson and Williamson 1999). There are clear links between contemporary research and colonial practices of studying Indigenous peoples and stealing cultural property and artifacts.

As a response to such ethical violations, and as part of reclaiming control over research, Indigenous peoples have developed a variety of ethical guidelines. In this context, ethics has been defined as a set of written and unwritten rules of conduct that express important social and cultural values (Castellano 2004). Indigenous organizations, funding agencies and groups of academics in Australia, Canada, New Zealand and the United States have published ethical guidelines to guide such research. In examining these guidelines, several common, overlapping themes emerge that are instructive to global health practitioners.

Research should uphold Indigenous self-determination

Indigenous scholar Castellano has noted, "Fundamental to the exercise of self-determination is the right of peoples to construct knowledge in accordance with self-determined definitions of what is real and what is valuable" (Castellano 2004: 102). Research should strengthen the ability of communities to define their own agenda around health improvement and to be able to take actions to implement this agenda. This includes upholding the right of communities to define who is and is not a member (Bartlett et al. 2007). Another aspect is respecting the right of Indigenous communities to govern and manage their own data. One example of how this right has been implemented in Canada is known as "ownership, control, access and possession of data" (OCAP) (Schnarch 2004). Ownership refers to the collective proprietary relationship that Indigenous communities have with their cultural knowledge, data and information. Control asserts that Indigenous peoples maintain authority over all aspects of research, including the conceptualization of the study question and hypothesis, the development and approval of the research design, data collection and management, data analysis, and the writing of the final report and its dissemination (Australian Government National Health and Medical Research Council 2003). The principle of access refers to the right of Indigenous communities to manage and make decisions about who can see and analyze data collected about them. Finally, possession refers to the ongoing retention of data by communities.

This ethical imperative to support the right of Indigenous peoples to determine their own knowledge processes has an inherent practicality: Indigenous involvement means that research knowledge is much more likely to be immediately relevant and useful to Indigenous communities. Indigenous self-determination of knowledge processes can therefore exemplify "intrinsic" knowledge translation processes.

Research should respect community customs and codes of practice

"Where the social, cultural or linguistic distance between the community and the researchers from outside the community is significant, the potential for misunderstanding is likewise significant" (Government of Canada Panel on Research Ethics 2008). Research should incorporate and value Indigenous worldviews. Community elders and holders of collective knowledge should be consulted and included as collaborators. At the same time, there should be an explicit plan to protect traditional knowledge, recognizing the troubling history of appropriation, commodification and unauthorized adaptation of Indigenous knowledge that has occurred. Academics should respect requests by Indigenous peoples to limit the publication of traditional knowledge.

Research should be centered around community engagement

Communities are groups of people who share an identity or interests and have the capacity to act or express themselves as collectives. Community engagement is "a process that establishes interaction between a researcher or research team, and the Aboriginal community... it signifies a collaborative relationship" (Government of Canada Panel on Research Ethics 2008). This goes beyond consultation to the involvement of community members and leaders at every stage of the research process, enhancing the authority of traditional governing bodies (Dickert and Sugarman 2005). This takes time and involves many steps (Lavery et al. 2010), including:

- Characterizing and building knowledge of the community, its diversity and changing needs
- Clarifying the purpose and goals of the research and understanding community perceptions and attitudes towards the research
- Establishing relationships with formal, informal and traditional leadership and building collaborative partnerships based on mutual respect (Tilburt and Kaptchuk 2008)
- Developing community assets and capacity
- Maximizing opportunities for stewardship, ownership and shared control by the community
- Respecting dissenting opinions and ensuring the opportunity to hear them
- Securing definitive permission/authority from the community

Research should be of social value

Research must be relevant to Indigenous communities and address needs and priorities identified by the community. Knowledge gained should have the potential to lead to new generalizable knowledge or improvements in health (Tilburt and Kaptchuk 2008). This relates to a broader concern for community welfare and contributes to the realization of collective rights. Importantly, research "should enhance [communities'] capacity to maintain their cultures, languages and identities" (Government of Canada Panel on Research Ethics 2008). Further, research should build capacity within the community by improving the infrastructure available and the knowledge and skills of individual community members.

Researchers should have the utmost respect for human biological materials

Given the importance placed on biological materials in many Indigenous cultures – and the troubling history of samples being collected and analyzed without community consent – the objectives, roles and responsibilities, and intended use of any samples collected should be clarified in a written research agreement before any work is undertaken. Following OCAP principles, the samples should be considered on loan to researchers and the rights to the samples should be kept by the community. Any secondary use of such samples would require community consent.

Interpretation and dissemination of research results

Indigenous communities should be the first to be informed of the results of any research. Community members should have the opportunity to participate in the data analysis, the writing of reports and presentations made, and should be able to validate or express concerns about any results before dissemination. Notably, discussions about intellectual property rights should occur well in advance of publication.

F) Conclusion

Fanon wrote that colonized societies may be able to "resolve problems to which Europe has not been able to find answers" (Fanon 1965: 6). Much can be learned from Indigenous values, which represent a powerful alternative centered on holism, a focus on community engagement, solidarity and social justice (WHO 2007b). "Values of collectivity, reciprocity, respect and reverence for Mother Earth, are crucial in the search for a transformed society where justice, equity, and sustainability will prevail" (Indigenous Peoples' Caucus 1999).

Global health practitioners can embody these values in their work to reduce health disparities (Horton 2006), particularly through a focus on addressing the social determinants of health. This should occur through affirming respect for all cultures, a focus on ecological renewal and sustainability, political empowerment, legal and institutional reform, enhancing economic prosperity, nurturing families and communities, and developing capacity within health and social systems (WHO 2007b).

References

Alfred, G.T. (2009) 'Colonialism and state dependency', *Journal of Aboriginal Health*, November: 42–60.

Anderson, I. et al. (2006) 'Indigenous health in Australia, New Zealand, and the Pacific', *Lancet*, 367(9524): 1775–85.

Australian Government National Health and Medical Research Council (2003) *Values and Ethics – Guidelines for Ethical Conduct in Aboriginal and Torres Strait Islander Health Research*. Canberra: Commonwealth of Australia.

Bartlett, J.G. et al. (2007) 'Identifying Indigenous peoples for health research in a global context: a review of perspectives and challenges', *International Journal of Circumpolar Health*, 66(4): 287–307.

Baskin, C. (2007) 'Aboriginal youth talk about structural determinants as the causes of their homelessness', *First Peoples Child & Family Review*, 3(3): 31–42.

Battiste, M. (2005) *Indigenous Knowledge: Foundation for First Nations*. University of Saskatchewan. www.viu.ca/integratedplanning/documents/IndegenousKnowledgePaper byMarieBattistecopy.pdf

Cancer Care Ontario (2008) *A Case Study Approach: Lessons Learned in Ontario: Aboriginal Tobacco Cessation*. Toronto: Aboriginal Cancer Care Unit, Cancer Care Ontario.

Castellano, M.B. (2004) 'Ethics of Aboriginal research', *Journal of Aboriginal Health*, January: 98–114.

Cunningham, C. and Stanley, F. (2003) 'Indigenous by definition, experience, or world view', *British Medical Journal*, 327(7412): 403–4.

Dickert, N. and Sugarman, J. (2005) 'Ethical goals of community consultation in research', *American Journal of Public Health*, 95(7): 1123–27.

Dodson, M. and Williamson, R. (1999) 'Indigenous peoples and the morality of the Human Genome Diversity Project', *Journal of Medical Ethics*, 25(2): 204–8.

Estey, E.A., Kmetic, A.M. and Reading, J. (2007) 'Innovative approaches in public health research: applying life course epidemiology to Aboriginal health research', *Canadian Journal of Public Health*, 98(6): 444–46.

Fanon, F. (1965) *The Wretched of the Earth*. New York: Grove Press.

Fantus, D. et al. (2009) 'Injury in First Nations communities in Ontario', *Canadian Journal of Public Health*, 100(4): 258–62.

Government of Canada Panel on Research Ethics (2008) *Tri-Council Policy Statement, Chapter 9: Research Involving Aboriginal Peoples*. Government of Canada Panel on Research Ethics. www.pre.ethics.gc.ca/eng/archives/draft-preliminaire/chapter9-chapitre9/

Harris, B., Russell, M. and Gockel, A. (2007) 'The impact of poverty on First Nations mothers attending a parenting program', *First Peoples Child and Family Review*, 3(3): 21–30.

Health Canada (2005) *First Nations Comparable Health Indicators*. Ottawa: Health Canada. www.hc-sc.gc.ca/fniah-spnia/diseases-maladies/2005-01_health-sante_indicat-eng.php

— (2010) *First Nations and Inuit Health: HIV and AIDS*. www.hc-sc.gc.ca/fniah-spnia/ diseases-maladies/aids-sida/index-eng.php

Horton, R. (2006) 'Indigenous peoples: time to act now for equity and health', *Lancet*, 367(9524): 1705–7.

Indigenous Peoples' Caucus (1999) *Indigenous Peoples' Seattle Declaration on the Occasion of the Third Ministerial Meeting of the World Trade Organization, 30 November–3 December 1999*. www.ldb.org/indi99.htm

Indigenous Physicians Association of Canada and Association of Faculties of Medicine of Canada (2008) *First Nations, Inuit, Metis Health Core Competencies: A Curriculum Framework for Undergraduate Medical Education*. Ottawa: Indigenous Physicians Association of Canada and Association of Faculties of Medicine of Canada.

International Work Group for Indigenous Affairs (n.d.) *Identification of Indigenous Peoples*. International Work Group for Indigenous Affairs. www.iwgia.org/culture-and-identity/identification-of-indigenous-peoples

Lavery, J.V. et al. (2010) 'Towards a framework for community engagement in global health research', *Trends in Parasitology*, 26(6): 279–83.

Ljunggren, D. (2009) 'Every G20 nation wants to be Canada, Stephen Harper insists', *The Calgary Herald*, 26 September.

Maina, F. (2003) 'Indigenous "insider" academics: educational research or advocacy?', *Canadian Journal of Native Studies*, 23(2): 207–26.

Matthews, J.D. (1997) 'Historical, social and biological understanding is needed to improve Aboriginal health', *Recent Advances in Microbiology*, 5: 257–334.

Michell, H. (2005). '"Nîhîthewâk of Reindeer Lake", Canada: Worldview, epistemology and relationships with the natural world', *Australian Journal of Indigenous Education*, 34: 33–43.

Montenegro, R.A. and Stephens, C. (2006) 'Indigenous health in Latin America and the Caribbean', *Lancet*, 367(9525): 1859–69.

Nettleton, C., Napolitano, D.A. and Stephens, C. (2007) *An Overview of Current Knowledge of the Social Determinants of Indigenous Health*. Geneva: World Health Organization, Commission on Social Determinants of Health.

Ohenjo, N. et al. (2006) 'Health of Indigenous people in Africa', *Lancet*, 367(9526): 1937–46.

Potvin, L. et al. (2003) 'Implementing participatory intervention and research in communities: lessons from the Kahnawake Schools Diabetes Prevention Project in Canada', *Social Science and Medicine*, 56(6): 1295–1305.

Reid, M. (2006) 'First Nations women works' speak, write and research back: child welfare and decolonizing stories', *First Peoples Child and Family Review*, 2(1): 21–40.

Royal Commission on Aboriginal Peoples (1996) *People to People, Nation to Nation: Highlights from the Report of the Royal Commission on Aboriginal Peoples*. Ottawa: Royal Commission on Aboriginal Peoples.

Said, E.W. (1979) *Orientalism*. New York: 1st Vintage Books.

— (1993) *Culture and Imperialism*. New York: Vintage Books.

Schnarch, B. (2004) 'Ownership, Control, Access and Possession (OCAP) or self-determination applied to research', *Journal of Aboriginal Health*, 1(1): 80–95.

Silver, J. (2007) *Unearthing Resistance: Aboriginal Women in the Lord Selkirk Housing Developments*. Ottawa: Canadian Centre for Policy Alternatives – Manitoba.

Smith, L.T. (1999) *Decolonizing Methodologies: Research and Indigenous Peoples*. New York: Zed Books.

Smylie, J. and Adomako, P. (eds) (2009) *Indigenous Children's Health Report: Health Assessment in Action*. Toronto: Center for Research on Inner City Health.

Smylie, J. and Anderson, M. (2006) 'Understanding the health of Indigenous peoples in Canada: key methodological and conceptual challenges', *Canadian Medical Association Journal*, 175(6): 602–5.

Smylie, J. et al. (2006) 'Indigenous health performance measurement systems in Canada, Australia, and New Zealand', *Lancet*, 367(9527): 2029–31.

Smylie, J. et al. (2011). *Our Health Counts: Urban Aboriginal Health Database Research Project – Community Report First Nations Adults and Children, City of Hamilton.* Hamilton: De Dwa Da Dehs Ney's Aboriginal Health Centre. www.stmichaelshospital.com/crich/our-health-counts-report.php

Stephens, C. et al. (2005) 'Indigenous peoples' health – why are they behind everyone, everywhere?', *Lancet*, 366(9479): 10–13.

— (2006) 'Disappearing, displaced, and undervalued: a call to action for Indigenous health worldwide', *Lancet*, 367(9527): 2019–28.

Ten Fingers, K. (2005) 'Rejecting, revitalizing, and reclaiming: First Nations work to set the direction of research and policy development', *Canadian Journal of Public Health*, 96(Suppl. 1): S60–63.

Tilburt, J.C. and Kaptchuk, T.J. (2008) 'Herbal medicine research and global health: an ethical analysis', *Bulletin of the World Health Organization*, 86(8): 594–99.

United Nations (2007) *United Nations Declaration on the Rights of Indigenous Peoples, 13 September 2007.* New York: United Nations.

— (2009) *State of the World's Indigenous Peoples.* New York: United Nations.

UN Permanent Forum on Indigenous Issues (n.d.) *About Us. Permanent Forum: Origin and Development.* United Nations Permanent Forum on Indigenous Issues. http://social.un.org/index/IndigenousPeoples/AboutUsMembers.aspx

University of Victoria Center for Aboriginal Health Research (2010) *Global Indigenous Health: An Opportunity for Canadian Leadership.* Victoria: Center for Aboriginal Health Research.

WHO (2007a) *Health of Indigenous Peoples Fact Sheet.* Geneva: World Health Organization. www.who.int/mediacentre/factsheets/fs326/en/index.html

— (2007b) 'Social determinants and Indigenous health: the international experience and its policy implications', report on socially prepared documents, presentations and discussion, in: *International Symposium on the Social Determinants of Indigenous Health, Adelaide, 29–30 April 2007.* Geneva: World Health Organization.

Wilmer, F. (1993) *The Indigenous Voice in World Politics: Since Time Immemorial.* Newbury Park: Sage.

PART II
Practice

7 Ethics and clinical work in global health*

Athanase Kiromera, Jane Philpott,
Sarah Marsh and Adrienne K. Chan

Objectives

- To highlight some of the key ethical considerations encountered in global health when working in a clinical setting
- To discuss the challenges clinical trainees face within global health

A) Introduction

Clinical work is perhaps the most common way in which health professionals engage in global health. This occurs in a variety of ways, including short- and long-term missions, work within humanitarian non-governmental organizations (NGOs) as volunteers or through long-term employment, and within public or private sector institutions as part of training initiatives and through bilateral exchange programs. Engaging in patient care is often seen as an opportunity to apply one's skills in a concrete and immediate way and to address the disparity seen in access to health services. However, concerns exist about the potential for negative repercussions when professionals from high-income countries (HIC) perform clinical duties in low- and middle-income countries (LMIC), not just for the patient, but also for her community, for the practitioner, and for the organization to which she belongs.

This chapter seeks to explore key ethical issues in global health clinical work through a series of cases based on our collective experiences as clinicians. We draw on the principles of the classic bioethics framework of Beauchamp and Childress (1989): beneficence (do good), nonmaleficence (do no harm), respect for individual autonomy

*The authors wish to acknowledge the contribution of case study content from Dr. Cheryl Hunchak, Global Health Emergency Medicine, University Health Network, University of Toronto, Canada.

and a commitment to justice. However, in order to explore some of the unique aspects of global health work, including cross-cultural understandings of health and issues of distributive justice within resource-limited settings, we also incorporate the framework of Pinto and Upshur (2009) that has been developed throughout this book: humility, introspection, solidarity and social justice (see Chapters 2 and 3).

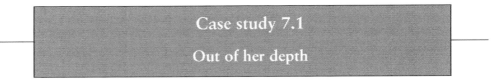

Case study 7.1

Out of her depth

Melanie was a first-year resident from Canada, doing a one-month elective in a rural hospital in Malawi. Before leaving Canada, Melanie completed a short pre-departure training course that was mandated by her program. She attended several lectures on working in low-resource settings and communicated with more senior trainees who had done similar electives. Melanie also contacted the physician who coordinated electives at the hosting hospital in Malawi and discussed her objectives for the rotation.

With a special interest in obstetrics and gynecology, the physician agreed to have her spend her time with clinicians and nurses in the Labor and Delivery ward during her placement. When Melanie arrived in Malawi she had a brief orientation by her supervisor and was introduced to the staff. She found the first few weeks difficult as all her interactions with patients took place in the local language, Chichewa. Melanie often felt guilty about being a burden to the clinician or nurse she was working with, as one of the staff always had to act as a translator. Most days she did not see a single patient who spoke English. Because of ongoing staff shortages, she was often not supervised. However, she learned to work independently and assist with many vaginal deliveries and Caesarean sections. She noted that the techniques employed were quite different from what she had seen in Canada.

Towards the end of her rotation, on a night while she was on call with a clinical officer, Melanie saw a woman who had been in labor for two days. The obstetrical nurse noted that the fetal heart rate was significantly decreased and conveyed that an urgent Caesarean section was needed. The clinical officer was called for several times but could not be reached. The nurse turned to Melanie and said, "You should do the C-section, otherwise this baby will die." Melanie was incredibly scared. She had never done a Caesarean alone and was worried that an attempt could kill both the woman and the infant. However, she felt that inaction could also cause the infant to die in utero and possibly harm the mother. Melanie told the nurse that she did not know how to do a Caesarean section on her own and encouraged her to call one of the other clinical officers, hoping that they would respond.

Reflective questions

1 How should a clinician respond when they are asked to perform a task that they do not feel competent doing? What factors would be important to consider?
2 With the potential for harm regardless of what Melanie does, how should she decide on what to do?
3 What are the possible long-term consequences for the patient, for Melanie and for the hospital if she does or does not perform the caesarean? What would happen if she does perform it, and there is a positive outcome?
4 Considering global health electives such as the one outlined, who benefits? Who bears the burden?
5 What factors influence the balance between service and learning in a global health setting?

B) Discussion of Case Study 7.1

This case illustrates a number of ethical issues, including concerns that are specific to trainees engaged in global health and concerns about exceeding one's capacity.

The number of trainees pursuing electives, international service learning and placements in LMIC under the banner of global health is large and growing (McKinley et al. 2008; Elit et al. 2011). Many trainees report facing significant ethical challenges that they were ill-prepared to face (Conard et al. 2006; Einterz 2008; Dowell and Merrylees 2009). A number of factors influence this, including the level of training of the student, their past experience with working in resource-limited settings, whether they speak the local language and have some understanding of the local context, if they have a local mentor and the duration of the experience (Torjesen et al. 1999; Niemantsverdriet et al. 2005; Federico et al. 2008). Pre-departure training appears to play some role in mitigating harm, and seemed to provide Melanie with some background and resources to employ when she was faced with this and other situations (Anderson et al. 2012).

This relates to the responsibilities of the sending and hosting institutions to trainees (Lancet 1993), a discussion that often does not take place. The scope of practice for each trainee should form part of memoranda of understanding and uphold local regulating bodies. Host institutions and local supervisors should ensure the student enters a safe environment that is appropriate for his or her level of skill and expectations, and should provide ongoing feedback and evaluation to trainees (White and Cauley 2006; Elit et al. 2011). Sending institutions should work to ensure trainees are prepared – including clinical skills and language training – and have clear learning objectives that fit within their course of study. They bear the ultimate responsibility for the actions of their trainees, regardless of their location. Further, sending institutions must work with host institutions to minimize the significant costs that outside trainees entail. This includes the time taken away from training local students, translation services and slowing the pace of clinics. The perverse situation whereby LMIC countries are indirectly subsidizing the training of HIC health professionals has been addressed in some organizations by providing a stipend to host institutions. Even better, perhaps, would be having trained faculty from the sending institution present to share the burden of teaching and to assist in building relationships and the establishment of true partnerships (see also Chapter 9).

The case clearly highlights a situation that was beyond Melanie's skills and experience, yet she needed to act. Clinical medicine often presents us with situations that must be dealt with at the time and decisions that cannot be deferred. Unfortunately, part of what structured the encounter is the assumption that Melanie – simply by being from a HIC – would know what to do (see Chapter 1). Appropriately, Melanie's first response was to show humility in recognizing that she could not do the Caesarean section alone. Adequate knowledge of one's level of training and the tasks that one can do independently or with supervision is crucial (Ackerman 2010). Melanie followed the principle of nonmaleficence, of particular importance for trainees who may have significant gaps in their clinical skills but may be under pressure to intervene given the dire nature of the situation. Importantly, this situation could have been prevented. Emergency caesarean sections on an obstetrical unit would not be uncommon. The staff shortages and high workload predictably led to a situation where Melanie was given unexpected responsibilities, putting the life of the patient at risk and causing significant distress to the trainee (Crump and Sugarman 2008).

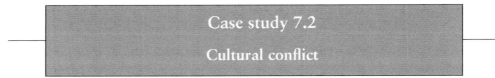

Case study 7.2

Cultural conflict

A young man is carried by his family into a busy emergency department of a large city hospital in East Africa. The young man has been in a motorcycle accident. He is unconscious, covered in vomit, and bleeding from his mouth and ears. Torsten, a visiting fellow from a HIC, determines that intubation is necessary. He calls out "Suction, please!" The head nurse runs for the lone suction machine in the department, which has just been used for another patient. New tubing and a plug are required. There is no outlet near the patient's bed so he is wheeled to the centre of the emergency department where the plug can reach a power source. It is discovered there is no adaptor and the head nurse rushes off to find one.

Gradually other items are gathered: Ambu bag, tubing, endotracheal tube, oral airway. Nurses are asked to rapidly bring together tape, intravenous (IV) lines and drugs. Slowly, an oxygen tank is brought from across the room. A visiting professor appears to review with Torsten the specifics of intubation while the patient receives oxygen. One pupil is becoming fixed and larger than the other, and he vomits. The clinical team scrambles to roll the patient on his side.

The suction is connected but the tubing is the calibre of an IV line and can't adequately clear his mouth. A stylet can't be located so the clinical team decides to do without. The laryngoscope blade arrives but the light is not working. A flashlight is produced.

Unaware of the resource situation around ventilators, Torsten speaks to the family about the need for intubation and asks if they will be willing to ventilate the patient manually until a ventilator becomes available. They agree. The drugs are given and the resident prepares to intubate. The flashlight is held over his shoulder. The height of the bed is non-adjustable and about eighteen inches lower than ideal. The airway is suctioned, the light repositioned. It is difficult to pass the tube without a stylet but he manages after several tries. The portable oxygen saturation probe reads 85 per cent. The Ambu bag is connected and soon the probe reads 98 per cent. The family is standing by, obviously worried. With the tube in place, they breathe a collective sigh of relief. The family begins to call around to collect the money for a CT scan, watching the rise and fall of the young man's chest.

It took forty-five minutes to gather half of the equipment required for a smooth intubation. The next challenge will be finding a ventilator, which Torsten now realizes may not be readily available. In the meantime, Torsten begins to express his frustration at the whole scene. He wonders why they can't keep the proper tubing with the suction equipment. He is angry about the way everything moved so slowly in the resuscitation process. At the same time, the head nurse remarks to her colleagues that these new visitors seem very demanding and they don't really understand the way things are usually done.

Reflective questions

1 Identify the sources of conflict in this scenario and why each participant appears to be dissatisfied with how it ended.
2 Why is the visiting fellow angry? What are the underlying assumptions to his emotions?
3 Could the resident have prepared better for working in this context? How?
4 What are the potential positive and negative consequences of the visiting fellow's work on the local health care providers?
5 How does decision-making happen in an emergency, and how should decisions be made about the goals of care?

C) Discussion of Case Study 7.2

This case raises a number of related ethical concerns, including cross-cultural competencies and concerns related to obtaining informed consent.

Important issues arise when one works in a new clinical setting and encounters different perspectives and expectations regarding the meaning of health, illness, treatment and the role of the health care system. It is not unusual for a newcomer to notice different approaches or priorities in a system with which they are not familiar. Torsten, similar to many HIC health professionals who work for a short period in an LMIC, describes these differences in the form of criticism. All too often this replicates a pattern whereby HIC professionals feel they know the best way to accomplish something. As an outsider, it may take many years properly to understand the reasons for the differences noted.

Cultural factors are clearly central. Much medical education scholarship in this area has focused on improving cultural sensitivity or awareness. In this conceptualization, the problem is a lack of exposure to the fact that people are different. Taking this further, achieving cultural competence is framed as addressing ignorance of other communities and peoples. However, this approach has been criticized for lumping people together and rarely examining the interplay between different identities. As an alternative based on critical pedagogy, insurgent multiculturalism provides opportunities to look at one's own biases, to challenge assumptions, to know people beyond labels, to confront the effects of power and privilege (and how life is lived without them), in order to develop a greater capacity for compassion and respect (Wear 2003). This deeper and more critical view of medical training is perhaps best suited to global health and achieving what has been called transnational competency (Koehn 2006).

It can be very difficult for a visiting trainee to understand why their clinical goals are different from their hosts'. However, it is important to make observations and ask questions in a manner that is respectful and non-judgemental. Skillful communication across cultures is an essential area of competence for all health care providers to achieve. An appreciation of different values and health care goals is also required.

Informed consent in LMIC can be complex. Even local health practitioners may struggle to obtain informed consent. The objective is to allow the patient to make an informed decision based on options that are reasonable for that person and appropriate given their context. Ultimately it is the patient who assigns weight to the risks and benefits and who makes the decision to proceed or not. Very often, patients do not truly understand their options and they may find explanations to be confusing. Working in LMIC may expose trainees to patients who do not know their rights. Patients might be afraid to challenge decisions, be too intimidated to ask questions, or be unaware about alternative options (Crump and Sugarman 2008; Hanson et al. 2011). Caring for such patients requires good communication skills, adequate language capabilities or the use of a translator. Furthermore, without an understanding of social and cultural norms it is difficult for students to truly obtain informed consent. The patient's community situation, family and level of education all have an impact on health and should be taken into consideration when developing a plan of care (Greannam 2003; Einterz 2008).

Sangita is working at a rural district referral hospital in Zimbabwe. Her responsibilities include managing the medical wards with fifty beds, as well as staffing the outpatient HIV and TB clinic. She is expected to be on call once every four nights, alternating with two general medical officers and the Chief Medical Officer.

Although the health infrastructure had been strong historically, with well-trained professional health staff, the health system is in the midst of extraordinary challenges. In addition to the significant "brain drain" that has occurred to neighboring countries, Europe and North America, there is currently a strike in the public sector. Due to the economic situation, there are persistent shortages of commodities (including commercial food supply and drugs), fuel shortages and electricity blackouts. The district hospital is run administratively by a missionary organization and so is not prioritized to receive a regular supply of medicines from the government based on their service agreement with the Ministry of Health and Social Welfare. Stocks at the hospital, as well as salary top-ups to support staff retention, are supported primarily by small private donations from charitable organizations in Canada and Europe, and from supplies brought in by volunteering physicians.

One night, Sangita's on call and is urgently asked to see a pediatric patient who was admitted to the hospital during the day. She has just finished admitting a twenty-five-year-old dehydrated, HIV-positive man who is on antiretroviral therapy (ART) and cotrimoxazole preventive therapy (CPT) and has a CD4 of 200 suggesting his immune system is quite compromised. He presented with fever, myalgia, headache and vomiting, and has a presumptive diagnosis of malaria, as his malaria smear is positive. After rehydrating the gentleman, she has asked the medicine nurse to see if there are any vials of IV quinine on any of the wards in the hospital.

Immediately after, a nurse has asked Sangita to come immediately because the child is seizing in the pediatric ward. A three-year-old girl was brought in by her mother after five days of a febrile illness and headache. She had been complaining of headache and nausea and was transferred to the referral hospital yesterday, when she started to develop decreased level of consciousness and jaundice. She was started on broad-spectrum oral antibiotics and sulfadoxine-pyremethamine plus chloroquine in a rural health post for possible malaria and sepsis of unknown origin. Upon arrival at the hospital, she was obtunded and so the clinical officer during the day started the child on IV antibiotics due to possible meningitis. The lumbar puncture results that came back look normal with zero white blood cells. Chemistry is not available. Gram stain and India ink are negative. The child's HIV status is unknown although the child's mother is HIV-positive and on antiretroviral therapy. Sangita assesses the child and is able to give her diazepam to stop the seizures, however she is extremely concerned that the child may have cerebral malaria.

The nurse from the medicine ward comes to find her and tells her that there is only enough IV quinine for a single individual. The only other antimalarials in hospital are oral sulfadoxine-pyramethamine and chloroquine, to both of which the fellow is certain there are high levels of *Plasmodium falciparum* resistance. Sangita knows from experience that she will be unable to obtain IV quinine from other health facilities or NGOs, due to the absence of fuel. When she assesses the child, her pupils are fixed and dilated and she is decerebrating; she strongly suspects the prognosis is poor due to anoxia. She decides to give the quinine to the adult male, who recovers and is discharged in a day, and palliate the child. The child dies in the morning.

Reflective questions

1   What are the key ethical principles that one considers when making decisions about limited resources? How are conflicts between principles addressed?
2   How would you approach this decision about who receives a potentially life-saving resource? What would be the factors that you would consider?
3   This scenario occurs in a certain context. Is there a role for health professionals in addressing the broader issue of social inequity? Is it a duty?

D) Discussion of Case Study 7.3

This case illustrates a scenario faced by many global health practitioners and the day-to-day reality of many health systems around the world. When two or more individuals require a limited resource, who should receive it? Theories may provide some guidance (see Chapter 2). At first glance, utilitarianism is intuitively appealing in making health resource allocation choices and seems to underpin the clinical decisions made by Sangita in this situation. Physicians make decisions like this every day when they allocate clinical resources or prioritize patients, whether it is triaging patients in an emergency room, or deciding on transfers of critically ill patients into intensive care unit beds. Decisions are made in clinical settings by finding a balance between the greatest need and also the potential for greatest benefit. The goal of achieving maximum good, whereby good is equivalent to health for the greatest number of people, seems to fit with our intuitive notions of justice for all (especially the marginalized) and our moral obligation. It seems to be a good thing to want what's best for human beings as a whole and also be concerned with public health outcomes for overall improvement of wellbeing.

The problem with consequentialism is that there is no moral obligation for the equal distribution of how interventions to improve public health are shared, which seems inherently unfair. The only moral obligation for a utilitarian is the greatest good for the greatest number of people, and as such, a utilitarian is not concerned at all with equal distribution of resources or how things are shared, merely with what increases the total good. Sangita's painful choice is a reminder of the choices that clinicians are forced to make that seem to go against the principles of justice, and highlights a physician's obligations to his or her patients that go above the pressing need of the immediate clinical dilemmas that we face in practice.

Apart from examining consequences, physician advocates should be concerned with the just and equal distribution of goods, because it is important that individuals are afforded the same benefit and burden, and fairness is to have equal treatment of all individuals in a just society, while minimizing in disparities in health. Sangita's obligations are not simply to following ethical principles around immediate decision-making around the case, but also in going further to address root causes.

Case study 7.4

Medical humanitarianism and ethics

Max has worked in Haiti for five years as a program coordinator for a social justice and health non-governmental organization. For over twenty years this organization has worked in partnership with the Ministère de la Santé Publique et de la Population (MSPP) to provide primary health services to the rural poor of central Haiti.

On January 12, 2010, the country experiences a massive earthquake near the capital, Port-au-Prince (PaP). At the time, Max is at the NGO's headquarters, sixty miles north of PaP. Eight days later, Max is sent to a large public hospital supported by his organization to help with coordinating the response. Earthquake victims have overwhelmed the hospital. There are over 200 patients requiring surgery, more than ninety with compound fractures and crush injuries. Much of the hospital staff is unaccounted for, assumed to be missing, searching for loved ones or involved in other emergency response efforts in PaP. A team of volunteer orthopedic and trauma surgeons, anesthesiologists, nurses and operating room (OR) technicians from the academic medical system of another country has been on site for several days with little accompaniment. The hospital is unaccustomed to foreign surgical teams, and Max has been sent to facilitate because integration of the short-term expatriate specialist teams has been a challenge.

The visiting team has reorganized the ORs and post-operative space to meet their needs, without much involvement of the existing staff. Foreign volunteers and local staff are working almost entirely independently, with little interaction or communication. The scene is chaotic and the hospital staff, expatriate volunteers, patients and family members are exhausted and increasingly frustrated and angry. Several patients have refused amputations from the volunteer team and have left the hospital.

Upon arrival, Max is immediately bombarded with complaints from all parties. The visiting team is working tirelessly, but quickly experiences both physical and emotional burnout. They are frustrated by the lack of infrastructure and their inability to communicate with local staff and patients. They perceive a lack of sense of urgency, difference in work ethic and lack of organization. They would like to run the OR twenty-four hours a day, but find no support from the Haitian surgical team and hospital administration. They are disturbed that patients are leaving the hospital rather than undergoing what they consider life-saving surgery to amputate limbs. They are concerned that they are unable to convey the appropriate information to patients and are therefore failing to do their job. They are also uncomfortable that the Haitian nurse-anesthetists are recommending regional versus general anesthetic, claiming that patients are requesting not to be put to sleep for fear that they will not wake up or that their limbs will be amputated without their consent.

The Haitian team is also demoralized. Most have lost friends and family members and many have lost their homes. There is a shortage of skilled providers to meet patient needs. The frequent explosions of anger and frustration directed at them by the visitors, and the expectation that the existing system needs to be changed, upset the local staff. They are opposed to operating the ORs twenty-four hours a day because of a severe shortage of skilled nurses to provide post-op care to critical patients. They voice particular concern around autonomy and informed consent with respect to amputations of crush-injured limbs. The visiting medical team seems unaware that rehabilitation services and limb prostheses are unavailable for most in Haiti. Local staff know that patients are terrified of amputation and feel that it might give them a life that they would rather not live as a burden to their community. Patients and their families express to Haitian staff that they feel that the care provided by the foreign physicians is substandard.

Max realizes that the conflict is reaching a boiling point which, if not resolved, will be harmful to patients and their immediate and future surgical and rehabilitation needs, and to the system, which will need the support and collaboration of multiple partners in order to provide services under the immense stress caused by this disaster for years to come.

Reflective questions

1 Why is conflict on teams with shared goals occurring? What is underlying these tensions?
2 What is the role of local perspectives? What happens when there is conflict between the views of the local population and the views of the outsider clinician?
3 In the setting of a humanitarian disaster, is there a moral obligation to ensure there is adequate post-operative care available as part of short-term medical relief?

E) Discussion of Case Study 7.4

The medical response to the earthquake in Haiti highlights key ethical issues common to humanitarian aid and well outlined in the literature (Hunt 2008). The earthquake catalyzed a rapid response from actors previously unengaged in medical humanitarian work, but whose skills were critically needed in the early response to the disaster. The catastrophic event also occurred in the setting of existing but now incapacitated physical and human resources for health infrastructure. In Haiti, socio-political factors that existed prior to the event also determined 'structured health risks' that the humanitarian crisis exacerbated (Pinto 2010; Chung 2012). Clearly the volume and urgency of needs in Haiti were elevated post-earthquake, which required health workers to work extremely long shifts. In settings of disaster relief, where expatriate teams and local teams work closely in a high-pressure situation, differences that exist around cultural frameworks in how health, wellness, disease and disability are understood and experienced can be exacerbated (Hunt 2011).

Specifically, carrying out multiple amputations highlighted the tension between local and foreign views of best practice (Etienne et al. 2011). The expatriate volunteers felt they were doing the right thing for patients, particularly given limited resources. Local staff had a different understanding of illness and disability, and were concerned about the long-term quality of life of patients. Barriers, not the least of which is language (Bjerneld et al. 2004), can prevent team members from responding to the cultural values and needs of patients and their understanding of disease. In Haiti, the loss of a limb appeared to be worse than death or dying because of the burden that amputees may be to their family and community. In spite of the clear short-term benefit, the patient perceives that they will likely become malnourished, maltreated and infected, may sustain further injury, and will face discrimination within the resource-stretched health care system, as well as encounter difficulties in procuring gainful employment. Many short-term surgical teams did not take into consideration that post-operative care would be a major issue, with very limited rehabilitation services and access to prosthetics compared with what one would expect in a resource-rich setting (Iezzoni and Ronan 2010; Landry et al. 2010).

This is not to suggest that a clinician should equate "first do no harm" with "first do nothing" (Morgan 2007). But it is important that "dominant principles sometimes need to be prioritized differently to be relevant to the context" (Hunt 2009), and the use of local role models is key. If unavailable, transnational actors such as Max may serve an important purpose. From an organizational perspective, imbalances of power that are already inherent in health care "hierarchy" are amplified in settings like Haiti post-earthquake. Pinto (2010) writes that the humanitarian impulse informing the international response may serve to reinforce further the historical relationship between wealthy countries and Haiti, and may fuel continued underdevelopment. The nature of organizations and individuals that choose to work in a vulnerable setting can easily, without critical self-reflection, amplify neocolonial power imbalances (Hunt 2011).

Finally, workers involved in humanitarian responses have an obligation to find and formalize consensus around policies, coordination and support to decrease ambiguity and expectations in these situations. Examples of post-event initiatives to address the concerns that arose from the Haiti earthquake include the development of "Consensus statements regarding the multidisciplinary care of limb amputation patients in disasters or humanitarian emergencies" by multiple stakeholders (Knowlton et al. 2011) to guide practitioners in similar situations in the future, as well as a proposal put forth by Médecins sans Frontières for the formation of an Emergency Surgery Coalition (ESC) of organizations with extensive experience in delivering care in humanitarian emergencies, which could deploy rapidly and be involved in pre-disaster preparation and training, inter-agency coordination and supply chain and logistics, and monitoring and evaluation post-disaster (Chu et al. 2011).

F) Conclusion

Adopting a critical approach to clinical work both before, during and after experiences is essential for practitioners to continue to work in resource-limited settings and in humanitarian crises. Taking the time to think about the complex ethical dimensions of working in these settings can prevent health workers from causing unnecessary harm, and also enhance relationships between health providers and their colleagues in these settings, as well as with patients.

References

Ackerman, L.K. (2010) 'The ethics of short-term international health electives in developing countries', *Annals of Behavioral Science and Medical Education*, 16(2): 40–43.

Anderson, K.C., Slatnik, M.A., Pereira, I., Cheung, E., Xu, K. and Brewer, T.F. (2012) 'Are we there yet? Preparing Canadian medical students for global health electives', *Academic Medicine*, 87(2): 206–9.

Beauchamp, T.L. and Childress, J.F. (1989) *Principles of Biomedical Ethics*, 3rd edn. New York, Oxford: Oxford University Press.

Bjerneld, M., Lindmark, G., Diskett, P. and Garrett, M.J. (2004) 'Perceptions of work in humanitarian assistance: interviews with returning Swedish health professionals', *Disaster Management and Response*, 2(4): 101–8.

Chu, K., Stokes, C., Trelles, M. and Ford, N. (2011) 'Improving effective surgical delivery in humanitarian disasters: lessons from Haiti', *PLoS Medicine*, 8(4): e1001025. doi: 10.1371/journal.pmed.1001025

Chung, R. (2012) 'A theoretical framework for a comprehensive approach to medical humanitarianism', *Public Health Ethics*, doi: 10.1093/phe/phs001

Conard, C.J., Kahn, M.J. and DeSalvo, K.B. (2006) 'Students' clinical experience in Africa: who are we helping?' *Virtual Mentor*, 8(12): 855–58.

Crump, J.A and Sugarman, J. (2008) 'Ethical considerations for short-term experiences by trainees in global health', *JAMA*, 300(12): 1456–58.

Dowell, J. and Merrylees, N. (2009) 'Electives: isn't time for a change?' *Medical Education*, 43(2): 121–26.

Einterz, E.M. (2008) 'The medical student elective in Africa: advice from the field', *Canadian Medical Association Journal*, 178(11): 1461–63.

Elit, L., Hunt, M., Redwood-Cambpell, L., Ranford, J., Adelson, N. and Schwartz, L. (2011) 'Ethical issues encountered by medical students during international electives', *Medical Education*, 45(7): 704–11.

Etienne, M., Powell, C. and Amundson, D. (2011) 'Healthcare ethics: the experience after the Haitian earthquake', *American Journal of Disaster Medicine*, 5(3): 141–47.

Federico, S.G., Zachar, P.A., Oravec, C.M., Mandler, T., Goldson, E. and Brown, J. (2008) 'A successful international child health elective', *Archives of Pediatrics & Adolescent Medicine*, 160: 191–96.

Greannam, T. (2003) 'A wolf in sheep's clothing: a closer look at medical tourism', *Medical Ethics*, 1(1): 5054.

Hanson L., Harms, S. and Plamodom, K. (2011) 'Undergraduate international electives: some ethical and pedagogical considerations', *Journal of Studies in International Education*, 15(2): 171–85.

Hunt, M.R. (2008) 'Ethics beyond borders: how health professionals experience ethics in humanitarian assistance and development work', *Developing World Bioethics*, 8(2): 59–69.

— (2009) 'Resources and constraints for addressing ethical issues in medical humanitarian work: experiences of expatriate healthcare professionals', *American Journal of Disaster Medicine*, 4(5): 261–71.

— (2011) 'Establishing moral bearings: ethics and expatriate health care professionals in humanitarian work', *Disasters*, 35(3): 606–22.

Iezzoni, L.I. and Ronan, L.J. (2010) 'Disability legacy of the Haitian earthquake', *Annals of Internal Medicine*, 152(12): 812–14.

Knowlton, L.M., Gosney, G.E., Chackungal, S. et al. (2012) 'Consensus statements regarding the multidisciplinary care of limb amputation patients in disasters or humanitarian emergencies: report of the 2011 Humanitarian Action Summit Surgical Working Group on amputations following disasters or conflict', *Prehospital and Disaster Medicine*, 26(6): 1–10.

Koehn, P.H. (2006) 'Globalization, migration health, and educational preparation for transnational medical encounters', *Globalization and Health*, 2: 2. doi: 10.1186/1744-8603-2-2

Lancet (1993) 'The overseas elective: purpose or picnic?', Commentary, *Lancet*, 342(8874): 753–54.

Landry, M.D., O'Connell, C., Tardif, G. and Burns, A. (2010) 'Post-earthquake Haiti: the critical role for rehabilitation services following a humanitarian crisis', *Disability and Rehabilitation*, 32(19): 1616–18.

McKinley, D., Williams, S., Norcini, J. et al. (2008) 'International Exchange Programs and US Medical Schools', *Academic Medicine*, 83: S53–57.

Morgan, M.A. (2007) 'Another view of "humanitarian ventures" and "fistula tourism"', *International Urogynecology Journal*, 18: 705–7.

Niemantsverdriet, S., van der Vleuten, C.P.M., Majoor, G.D. and Scherpbier, A.J.J.A. (2005) 'An explorative study into learning on international traineeships: experiential learning processes dominate', *Medical Education*, 39: 1236–42.

Pinto, A.D. (2010) 'Denaturalizing "natural" disasters: Haiti's earthquake and the humanitarian impulse', *Open Medicine*, 4(4). www.openmedicine.ca/article/view/407/364

Pinto, A.D and Upshur, R.E.G. (2009) 'Global health ethics for students', *Developing World Bioethics*, 9(1): 1–10.

Suchdev, P., Ahrens, K., Click, E., Macklin, L., Evangelista, D. and Graham, E. (2007) 'A model for sustainable short-term international medical trips', *Ambulatory Pediatrics*, 7: 317–320.

Torjesen, K., Mandalakas, A., Kahn, R. and Duncan, B. (1999) 'International child health electives for paediatric residents', *Archives of Pediatrics & Adolescent Medicine*, 153: 1297–1302.

Wear, D. (2003) 'Insurgent multiculturalism: rethinking how and why we teach culture in medical education', *Academic Medicine* 78: 549–54.

White, M.T. and Cauley, K.L. (2006) 'A caution against medical students' tourism', *American Medical Association Journal of Ethics*, 8(12): 851–54.

Wimmers, P.F., Schmidt, H.G. and Splinter, T.A.W. (2006) 'Influence of clerkship experiences on clinical competence', *Medical Education*, 40: 450–58.

Further reading

Bhat, S. (2008) 'Ethical coherency when medical students work abroad', *Lancet*, 372: 1133–34.

Crump, J.A., Sugarman, J. and Barry, M. (2010) 'Ethics and best practice guidelines for training experiences in global health', *American Journal of Tropical Medicine and Hygiene*, 83(6): 1178–82.

Hardcastle, T.C. (2008) 'Ethics of surgical training in developing countries', *World Journal of Surgery*, 32: 1562.

Kingham, T.P., Muyco, A. and Kushner, A. (2009) 'Surgical elective in a developing country: ethics and utility', *Journal of Surgical Education*, 66: 59–62.

Mutchnick, I.S., Moyer, C.A. and Stern, D.T. (2003) 'Expanding the boundaries of medical education: evidence for cross-cultural exchanges' *Academic Medicine*, 78(10): 1–5.

Radstone, S.J.J. (2005) 'Practicing on the poor? Healthcare workers' beliefs about the role of medical students during their electives', *Journal of Medical Ethics*, 31: 109–10.

Ethical challenges in global health research

Ghaiath Hussein and Ross E.G. Upshur

Objectives

- To discuss the ethical principles underlying global health research
- To discuss the importance of community engagement and respect for local community process in global health research

A) Introduction

It is well recognized that health research is becoming more "globalized." While the large majority of clinical trials are led by teams based in high-income countries (HIC), health research now takes place in many low- and middle-income countries (LMIC). For example, health research infrastructure is rapidly developing in India, South Africa and Brazil. In a recent study, twenty-four of the twenty-five countries demonstrating the fastest growth in clinical trial sites were in emerging economies (Thiers et al. 2008). In parallel to the increased capacity for research, ethical review and oversight of this research is growing, but has not kept pace. As a report in the *British Medical Journal* noted:

> ...of the 100,000 clinical trials carried out around the world each year, some 10 per cent occur in developing countries, where patients are readily available, regulatory requirements are less strict, and costs are lower. By 2010 European and US drug companies are expected to spend $1.5bn (£0.8bn; €1.1bn) on trials in India alone. However, many developing countries, especially in Africa, do not have the logistical support, financial resources, or trained personnel to establish effective ethical committees or to supervise the research being carried out among their citizens.
>
> (Watson 2007: 1706).

The emergence of interest in global health research is tied to issues related to the conduct of certain trials in LMICs. Considerable controversy arose over placebo controlled trials in Africa, particularly the ACTG 076 trial to prevent mother-to-child transmission of HIV (Angell 1997). Some argued that using placebos when an established effective intervention was available, was unethical because it subordinated the welfare of participants to the goals of science. Others argued that placebo controlled trials were justified on the basis that participants were unlikely to be able to access effective preventive therapy in the location where the studies were being conducted. Furthermore, such trials presented the most expeditious means of determining whether such therapy was feasible in comparison with the local standard of care (Lurie and Wolfe 2007).

Global health research also raises issues concerning global justice, what constitutes fair benefits to individuals and communities participating in research, individual-level informed consent in communally based societies, and the importance of community engagement in health research. It has stimulated efforts to build capacity for ethical oversight in LMICs through training and educational programs.

The extent of the ethical challenges posed by global health, particularly in light of the discovery of unethical studies of syphilis transmission in Guatemala, prompted President Obama to direct the Presidential Advisory Committee to examine the current status of ethical standards of global health research. The report, Moral Science, outlines several key challenges that researchers may face in the conduct of global health research (Presidential Commission for the Study of Bioethical Issues 2011).

In this chapter, we will provide a brief historical introduction to the evolution of research ethics, outline its key principles and provide a framework for global health research, and discuss the importance of securing local review. The specific focus will be on contextual issues arising from research involving communities in LMICs that emphasize the importance of community engagement, particularly on research involving human subjects. Thus we will not, in this chapter, address ethical issues involved in population-based research. Also, we will not discuss the particular challenges raised by research in humanitarian responses.

B) Historical background to the ethical oversight of research

Modern research ethics has its origins in the Nuremburg trials, which took place shortly after the end of World War II. At these trials, it came to light that medical doctors subjected non-consenting humans to a variety of experiments, the vast majority having no scientific merit. These experiments inflicted untold suffering and death on those involved. As a result of the trials, the Nuremburg code enshrined the importance of voluntary consent as a *sine qua non* of any research involving human participants. The German and Japanese experiments were not isolated incidents. The recognition that health research in humans poses risks and that these risks were often not well communicated to participants was also apparent.

In subsequent decades, attention to ethical aspects of human subjects research increased. In 1964, the World Medical Association issued the Declaration of Helsinki as "a statement of ethical principles for medical research involving human subjects, including research on identifiable human material and data" (World Medical Association 1964). Henry Beecher also published an influential paper in 1966 that outlined ethical flaws in a number of studies (Beecher 1966). In the early 1970s, in the United States, the Tuskegee syphilis studies were exposed, where African American men infected with syphilis were studied long after it was established that penicillin was a safe and effective treatment. Beecher's paper and the Tuskegee revelations were influential in the creation of the Presidential Commission that created the Belmont Report. The Belmont Report identified three core ethical principles: respect for persons, beneficence, and justice as fundamental to research on human subjects (National Commission for the Protection of Human Subjects of Biomedical and Behavioral Research 1979).

There are now a wide range of guidance documents on ethical standards in research. A list of selected guidelines can be found at the end of this chapter. There are many structural similarities to these varied guidelines, but, more importantly, there is considerable variability and lack of harmonization across the globe. Greater efforts at consistency in guideline documents and in research ethics review is a major focus of current efforts in global health research.

C) Principles of research ethics

The ethical requirements for clinical research contained in the many guideline documents have been admirably summarized by Emanuel et al. (2000). Additional considerations for research in LMICs were added in 2004, emphasizing the importance of building collaborative partnerships (Emanuel et al. 2004). The principles have been adapted by the international humanitarian organization Médecins Sans Frontières as a guidance document for researchers designing studies, and by its ethics review board to assess the quality of the research (Schopper et al. 2009). These are outlined in Table 8.1.

Core to ethical research, regardless of where the research takes place, are concerns for the scientific validity and social value of the research. Poorly designed research will bring no benefit to humanity, squanders scarce resources and may place participants at needless risk. The criterion of social value directs researchers to be sensitive to the needs of populations. Fair subject selection and consideration of the balance of harms and benefits will reduce exploitation.

With respect to the avoidance of exploitation, research in LMICs directs research teams to think very carefully about ancillary care obligations. Research studies, particularly clinical trials, are designed to answer a specific hypothesis about the effects of particular interventions. Enrolled research subjects and the communities in which they live may have substantial unmet health needs, outside the scope of the research project, that will raise questions for researchers regarding the extent of their obligation to provide care. The studied communities may lack necessary services such as drinking water, basic health care or trained health care providers. Communities may expect international researchers to provide them the services they lack.

Table 8.1 Ethics framework for medical research, Médecins Sans Frontières

Principles	*Benchmarks*
Collaborative partnership	• Engage in partnership with national and/or international research institutions as relevant and appropriate. • Collaborate with local and national researchers and health policy-makers to determine the importance of health problems; assess the value of the research; plan, conduct and oversee the research; and integrate the results of the research into the health system as relevant and appropriate. • Respect the community's values, culture, traditions and social practices. • Involve the community in which the study takes place (the 'study community') through a consultative process in designing the research, in its implementation (advice on problems occurring during study, feedback of intermediate results) and in assessing how research results may be made beneficial.* • Contribute to developing the capacity for researchers and health policy-makers to become full and equal partners in the research enterprise where possible. • Share fairly the financial and other rewards of the research where possible.

Social value	• Specify the beneficiaries of the research.
	
	• Assess the importance of the health problems being investigated and the prospect of value of the research for the beneficiaries.
	
	• Devise and implement mechanisms to enhance the social value of the research by:
	
	  – disseminating the knowledge gained locally, nationally, regionally and internationally
	
	  – making drugs or interventions tested and found to be effective available to the study community through advocacy, by involving policy-makers from the start, and by staying long enough after research ends to ensure its application where possible.
	
	• Prevent supplanting the extant health system infrastructure and services.

Table 8.1 Continued

Principles	Benchmarks
Scientific validity	• Ensure the scientific design of the research realizes social value for the primary beneficiaries of the research. • Ensure the scientific design realizes the scientific objectives while guaranteeing research participants the health care interventions to which they are entitled (this includes a sample size sufficient to reach objectives). • Ensure the research study is feasible given the social, political and cultural environment and with sustainable improvements in the local health care and physical infrastructure.
Fair selection of study population	• Select the study population to ensure scientific validity of the research. • Select the study population to minimize risks of the research. • Formulate clear inclusion and exclusion criteria. • Identify and protect vulnerable populations.
Favorable harm–benefit ratio	• Assess the potential harms and benefits of the research to the study participants. • Assess the harm–benefit ratio for the community. • Involve the community in assessing potential harms and benefits for study participants and the community at large.

Informed consent	• Involve the study community in establishing appropriate recruitment procedures and incentives for the participants.
	
	• Ensure consent procedures are acceptable within the study community (may include supplementary community and familial consent procedures).
	
	• Ensure the method of informed consent (written versus oral) is appropriate for the study while respecting a study participant's right to be fully informed of all implications of their study enrolment.
	
	• Disclose information in culturally and linguistically appropriate formats. This implies that:
	  – any information given during the informed consent process must be pre-tested with people of a similar cultural and educational background as potential study participants
	  – the information provided on the consent form must be in simple language, avoiding technical terms

Table 8.1 Continued

Principles	Benchmarks
Informed consent (continued)	– the consent form must be translated into the local language and then back-translated into the 'international' language used to verify the accuracy of the translation – consent is obtained in culturally and linguistically appropriate forms** and mistakes corrected. • Ensure participants fully comprehend the research objectives and procedures. If needed, the person should have time to discuss the information received with members of the community or family before deciding on consent. In addition, community information or 'schooling' on the research to be done, and on the purpose and process of seeking informed consent, will raise pre-enrolment awareness and help people decide if they want to participate. • Obtain consent in culturally and linguistically appropriate formats.** • Ensure potential participants are free to refuse or withdraw from the research at any stage without penalty.

*'Community' can be described in many different ways. Most commonly, community is described as a geographical, functional or socio-cultural entity with characteristics such as shared interests and experiences, values, common fate or cultural affinity. Sometimes a community is already organized, for example in the form of village committees. However, care should be taken regarding their real capacity to represent the community. In addition, official community groups can be part of government, be repressive and coercive and deny human rights, severely interfering with the voluntary nature of participation. In some conflict-ridden environments, the social structure has been destroyed. In these contexts, it must be carefully explored who best represents the interests of the population.

If it is not possible to have a well functioning community body throughout the research process, at a minimum the community must be consulted during the planning stage of the research, consulted on an *ad hoc* basis while the research is being done, and informed about the results in a structured manner at the end of the research. It is not enough to carry out this dialogue by consulting local staff, as they may not really represent the community. One option would be to add a few current or past patients to the group planning the study to ensure the objectives, approach, etc., are adequate and adapted to the local context.

**In some settings, participants have refused to sign a consent form. Signing a consent form is not mandatory, but serves as a back-up proof for the principal investigator. If a person refuses to sign, but gives oral consent, the researcher should keep a written record that the patient has been informed, has understood and agreed to participate, but has refused to sign.

Researchers need to be clear from the very beginning about what they intend to do and exactly what "services" they may be able to provide. They should emphasize that these services are temporary, and that the community may need to work on making them more sustainable. Whether there is a moral duty on international researchers to help the studied communities has been debated in the literature (London 2005; Hawkins and Emanuel 2008). What researchers are capable of providing should be anticipated in advance, and an agreed-upon strategy with the community should be negotiated.

Lavery and colleagues have created a series of case studies with commentaries that illustrate the nuances of the application of ethical principles in actual research in LMICs (Lavery et al. 2007). It is important to note, as per Chapter 3, that there will inevitably be disagreement about how the principles should best be weighed. As noted above, there is still much work to be done to explicate more fully the extent of duties and obligations of researchers to individuals and communities involved in research. Judgment will always be required. However, Table 8.1 provides a framework that articulates the relevant, non-ignorable ethical considerations. As Emanuel et al. (2004) write:

> Disagreement on the balancing of the various benchmarks does not necessarily make one assessment ethical and the other unethical. Rather, it may reflect different but legitimate ways of resolving competing ethical claims. In fact, this framework can help narrow disagreements and elucidate the different underlying views.
>
> (Emanuel et al. 2004: 936)

D) Contextual considerations in research in LMICs

Research is more than just its conduct. Research affects, and is affected by, the context in which it is conducted. It is crucial for the researcher to be aware of the context in which her research is being conducted to avoid unnecessary risks, delays, or even cancellation of the whole study.

The importance of receiving local ethical review

Researchers must be aware of local research ethics boards and secure approvals before the commencement of research. This may mean a substantial amount of pre-departure preparation, as approval from the sponsoring organization or university may be required as well. It is the responsibility of the researcher to be aware of all regulations and permissions well in advance of commencement of the research. Seeking ethical approval from the local authorities, or ethics review committees, if present, may be seen by researchers as a bureaucratic step to get the job done. In fact, it may be so, but it serves another important contribution to sustainable development. If the local health authorities are being asked frequently for ethical approval of research proposals and not just administrative approval, this would raise their awareness of the importance of establishing an ethics review body, or activate it if it is already there. It is quite well established in the literature that most LMICs have reduced capacity to review and approve research (Glickman et al. 2009). Unfortunately, this situation has been abused by some international researchers and companies to conduct clinical trials on vulnerable people without proper consent or proper research oversight.

The importance of community engagement

Community engagement is increasingly recognized as an essential component of research in LMICs (Tindana et al. 2007). The recent report of the Presidential Commission for the Study of Bioethical Issues (2011) listed as one of its fourteen recommendations the need to promote community engagement. As yet, there are no agreed-upon standards for the optimal means by which researchers should engage communities. The ethical basis of community engagement lies in respect for communities and their cultures. It seeks to create an ongoing dialogue between communities and researchers. Furthermore, it should allow for the integration of "community norms, beliefs, customs, and cultural sensitivities into research activities" (Presidential Commission for the Study of Bioethical Issues 2011: 11). Tindana et al. (2007) have identified the following goals for community engagement:

- To ensure the relevance of research
- To assess whether relevant research is culturally and practically acceptable in the context it is intended
- To ensure that community disruption is minimized, e.g. avoiding the displacement of medical staff from pressing local needs
- To avoid exploitation by ensuring fair distribution of the benefits of research
- To take into account the ethical hazards that may be part of the social, economic and political landscape of the community

An important dimension of community engagement is the return of the results of research (see also OCAP principles discussed in Chapter 6). If research is to contribute to social justice, the body of knowledge created should be utilized for the benefit of the people. This contribution is never accomplished until the results of the research conducted are shared with relevant stakeholders. The main focus of many researchers is to share their research with their professional colleagues through conferences and peer-reviewed publications. The studied communities are less frequently thought about, especially if we consider that these communities are far away from the researcher who has conducted the research for a purpose, which is usually fulfilling an academic or a professional commitment. However, it could be argued that there is an ethical obligation on the researcher to share the results of the research with those who were studied. First, this is usually a part of the consent given by the research participant, and it is a logical expectation of the people who were studied. This should be considered as part of the collaborative partnership. Studied populations expect some benefit from their contribution to research, though they may expect tangible results such as better services; sharing the results is the least the researcher can provide to the studied communities.

There may be technical and ethical issues attached to this duty. Technically, researchers may have signed contracts with their funding agencies or the academic institutes that prohibit them from sharing any results without prior written permission from the sponsors. There are also issues related to how to share the results, and with whom. Are they best shared with the local health authorities, which will make better, wider-scale use of the results, or with community leaders, or with individual participants?

Practical approaches to sharing of results with the communities may include the following.

- Prior to the research, the researcher should include the data-sharing plan and have it approved by the research funders or sponsors. This plan should be clear about which results will be shared, when, with whom, and how.
- The consent should be clear about the sharing of results, even in cases where the researcher will not be able to share the results with individual participants or even community leaders. Participants should be aware of this, and should approve waiving their right to know the results.
- The researcher should collect the contact details of the local health authorities relevant to the area of research, the leaders of the studied communities, and the individual participants. The latter should not be part of the data-collection tool unless needed methodologically.
- Researchers do not have to share the results by themselves. This could be done through local leaders or NGOs working in the studied community. However, they should ensure the necessary confidentiality of this information, especially if data are identifiable.
- The inclusion of local co-investigators is usually advisable, and sometimes required by some countries. One of their tasks is to share the results with their communities in a way that is culturally appropriate.

Informed consent

Informed consent remains an important element of any research involving human subjects. For consent to participate in research to be ethically valid, it needs to be obtained from a person who is competent to respond freely and voluntarily after being fully informed about the relevant information related to the study in a language that she or he understands. The participant should have been given the chance to ask questions and have them answered clearly. Usually, but not necessarily, consent is obtained in writing and signed by the participant.

Implementation of the standards of consent to research by international researchers in the setting of LMICs is challenged by a number of factors. First, international researchers frequently have little or no knowledge about the country in which the research is conducted. This may lead researchers to seek translation of the consent forms and the data collection tools, especially questionnaires. The use of translators itself poses a set of ethical issues, including the extent of precision of the translation – to what extent the participant was really informed and the confidentiality of the information given by the participants, especially in smaller, rural communities where most people are relatives.

Second, the relatively higher rates of illiteracy among vulnerable groups and in rural areas where there is less access to education, among other basic services, makes it harder for participants to comprehend the translated consent. Particular efforts may be required to assure comprehension. Another important cultural factor that would affect obtaining consent is related to signing forms. Being asked to place one's signature on papers brought by strangers is treated by suspicion by many cultures that have suffered from experiences with fraud.

Third, consent may be hard to obtain because of language barriers and the strong family hierarchy that may be dominated by male members of the family. Addressing the role of the community leader or head of household in the decision of a potential participant to participate (or not) should be managed delicately to avoid unintentional offense to the leader and to ensure the rights of the participant are respected. If a man tells his wife or daughter to participate in a research study, you may still ask her in private if she really wants to take part. The researcher should reassure her that whatever she decides will not be conveyed to the head of the household.

Fourth, one must be careful and thoughtful about the use of incentives. Researchers need to avoid direct cash payments, unless justified by compensation for lost working hours and travel costs. This is not the norm in many Western countries, where participants are paid at the end of the research. However, in many LMICs people will volunteer for research and may even feel offended if they are offered payment for something that is to benefit the community.

Fifth, access to communities may rely on some form of community consent, or assent that may be granted only by the community leader(s). Researchers will need their assistance for official permissions or approvals required for research.

For international researchers, overcoming all these factors when obtaining consent in the context of LMICs is not easy; however, some practical advice may include the following.

- Have the consent forms and other data-collection tools (e.g. questionnaires) translated and back-translated by a colleague of the same country in the researcher's home institution before starting the study.
- Recruitment of translators and data collectors from the studied community should be preceded by proper training on consent and data-collection tools.
- A very clear and strict confidentiality agreement should be attached and signed by local data collectors when signing the research contract.
- Prior to data collection, the translated consent and questionnaire should be piloted with some lay members of the population to assess their appropriateness.
- If participants refuse to sign the consent, it may be useful to give them time to consult the community leader or anyone they trust. Providing them a copy of the consent with the researcher's contacts and affiliations would be reassuring.
- Train better-educated community members as data collectors, focused not only on the methodology but more importantly on ethical issues, especially those related to confidentiality.

Respect for communities: social structure, political and security considerations

Southern hemisphere communities may embody binding sets of family and tribal values. There may be a strong family and tribal hierarchy, where older persons are given dominant roles in decision-making. Although this picture is gradually diminishing due to the Westernization and industrialization of many of these communities, many people still retain these values.

Researchers may need to be wary of the potential influence of community leaders who may insist on having particular persons or households selected. Researchers need to talk to the community leaders and explain to them in simple terms what sampling is, why it is needed, and how it is done. It is important to explain that selected members or households will not gain extra benefit from such involvement, apart from the general benefit for the community.

Many LMICs have experienced political instability due to historic and contemporary interference by external forces and struggles over power and resources by internal forces (Hussein 2009). In such environments, where people are less free to share their opinions and concerns, community members may be hesitant to express themselves. Moreover, such communities may become polarized and divided because of competing political allegiances. Tensions between groups may become violent, especially during times of transition.

Access to the study area may be restricted. This may either delay the start of the research or adversely affect sampling. Researchers should plan for such instances when they know about any political or security instability in their suggested research area. Team members may be at increased risk and this could lead to serious implications for the progress of the research. Data collectors may be abducted or seriously threatened if they enter the research community at the wrong time or by the wrong route. Depending on the anticipated severity of the condition, the researcher needs to justify imposing such a risk on herself and on the research team. The team needs to have an evacuation plan in place if things become unstable. Data collectors should be informed of this and other contingency plans.

Many of the above-mentioned ways of conducting research in global health seem to be beyond the scope of the individual researcher. However, there are some practical approaches that could be taken by individual researchers before, during and after the conduct of research.

E) A checklist for researchers

Before conducting research

- The researcher should choose research questions that are relevant to the studied population. This would lead to the results being more usable at the end of the study in assisting the local development of the studied community. Research that is of high social value will support the building of collaborative partnerships.

- The researcher should have a local co-investigator(s) in the project. This will help local researchers build, or improve their capacity to conduct research.
- Prior communication with the studied communities before the start of the study has logistical, technical and ethical significance. Logistically, it sets the stage for easy access to the community to be studied, which is technically important to improve sampling, and to be more ethically fair. This communication can be utilized to provide some education about the importance of research in general, not only the intended study. This would raise the awareness of communities about the importance of research, and make it easier for the researchers to be accepted.
- Researchers should plan in advance what benefits can and will be shared with the studied communities. The concept of benefit should go beyond traditional, product-oriented benefits to more sustainable benefits. This would fulfill the requirement of fair subject selection and address issues related to harm and benefit.
- Consent issues should be addressed in terms of cultural appropriateness and accuracy of translation.

During the conduct of research

- The study should include a training component, where local data collectors develop their capacities in data collection and beyond. This would reinforce collaborative partnerships.
- The research should include training of local co-investigators, not only on competencies needed to achieve the particular project, but to include a wider scope of relevant skills and competencies.
- The research can also include training and/or health education components for the studied communities. This is a sustainable benefit from which the whole community benefits, not only those involved in the study.
- Obtaining consent may seem to be only an ethical (or regulatory) prerequisite for research. In reality, it can serve to be much more. Taking proper consents includes sharing of knowledge as well as asking questions. The exposure of the people to this small element of democracy will help them become empowered by establishing a trend of having the right to ask questions and to have them answered clearly. Moreover, the people may be practicing their right to object or to say no for the first time in their lives. Only a free community can have truly sustainable development.

After the end of research

- Research results and recommendations should be shared, especially results that can be utilized within the contexts of the studied communities.
- Communication with local researchers, health authorities and community leaders should be maintained.
- Colleagues at one's home institution may be encouraged to conduct further research and to join the existing collaboration.

- Proper care or referral to better health facilities may be offered for participants who were found to have diseases requiring special care.
- Researchers can act as advocates for the causes related to health research in LMICs.

F) Conclusion

In this chapter we have argued for the importance of researchers in global health understanding their ethical duties and responsibilities. They must be aware of international, national and local guidelines and regulations regarding the conduct of their proposed research. The process of securing appropriate and necessary approvals is vital for the ethical conduct of research. It is essential that researchers know as much as possible in advance about the context in which they will be conducting research. Community engagement and collaborative partnerships are vital components of the research process, as is discussing and negotiating benefit-sharing and the return of results. Ethically sound research is the best research, and is rewarding to both researchers and participants.

References

Angell, M. (1997) 'The ethics of clinical research in the developing world', *New England Journal of Medicine*, 337: 847–49.

Beecher, H. (1966) 'Ethics and clinical research', *New England Journal of Medicine*, 274: 1354–60.

Emanuel, E., Wendler, D. and Grady, C. (2000) 'What makes clinical research ethical?', *Journal of the American Medical Association*, 283(20): 2701–2.

Emanuel, E. et al. (2004) 'What makes clinical research in developing world ethical? The benchmarks of ethical research', *Journal of Infectious Disease*, 189(5): 930–37.

Glickman, S. et al. (2009) 'Ethical and scientific implications of the globalization of clinical research', *New England Journal of Medicine*, 360: 816–23.

Hawkins, J. and Emanuel, E.J. (eds) (2008) *Exploitation and Developing Countries: The Ethics of Clinical Research*. Princeton: Princeton University Press.

Hussein, G. (2009) 'Democracy: the forgotten challenge for bioethics in the developing countries', *BMC Medical Ethics*, 10(3).

Lavery, J.V. et al. (2007) *Ethical Issues in International Biomedical Research: A Casebook*. New York: Oxford University Press.

London, A. (2005) 'Justice and the human development approach to international research', *Hastings Centre Report*, 34: 24–37.

Lurie, P. and Wolfe, S. (1997) 'Unethical trials of interventions to reduce perinatal transmission of the human immunodeficiency virus in developing countries', *New England Journal of Medicine*, 337: 853–56.

National Commission for the Protection of Human Subjects of Biomedical and Behavioral Research (1979) *The Belmont Report: Ethical Principles and Guidelines for the Protection of Human Subjects of Research*. Bethesda, MD: National Institutes of Health. http://ohsr.od.nih.gov/guidelines/belmont.html

Presidential Commission for the Study of Bioethical Issues (2011) *Moral Science: Protecting Participants in Human Subjects Research*. http://bioethics.gov/cms/sites/default/files/Moral%20Science%20%28Updated%202012%29_0.pdf

Schopper, D. et al. (2009) 'Research ethics review in humanitarian contexts: the experience of the independent ethics review board of Médecins Sans Frontières', *PLoS Medicine*, 6(7).

Thiers, F.A. et al. (2008) 'Trends in the globalization of clinical trials', *Nature Reviews Drug Discovery*, 7: 13–14.

Tindana, P.O. et al. (2007) 'Grand challenges in global health: community engagement in research in developing countries', *PLoS Medicine*, 4(9).

Watson, R. (2007) 'Developing world needs stronger research guidelines', *British Medical Journal*, 334(7603): 1076.

World Medical Association (1964) *WMA Declaration of Helsinki – Ethical Principles for Medical Research involving Human Subjects*. World Medical Association. www.wma.net/en/30publications/10policies/b3/

Resources

General guidelines

Canada – Tricouncil Policy Statement – Ethical Conduct for Research Involving Humans: www.pre.ethics.gc.ca/eng/policy-politique/initiatives/tcps2-eptc2/Default/

Council for International Organizations of Medical Sciences: www.cioms.ch/publications/guidelines/guidelines_nov_2002_blurb.htm

Declaration of Helsinki: www.wma.net/en/30publications/10policies/b3/

India Council for Medical Research, Ethical Guidelines for Biomedical Research on Human Participants: http://icmr.nic.in/ethical_guidelines.pdf

Nuffield Council on Bioethics – Research in Developing Countries: www.nuffieldbioethics.org/research-developing-countries-follow

South Africa – Medical Research Council: www.mrc.ac.za/ethics/ethics.htm

World Health Organization – WHO Research Ethics: www.who.int/ethics/research/en

9

Ethical considerations of global health partnerships*

Jill Murphy, Victor R. Neufeld,
Demissie Habte, Abraham Aseffa,
Kaosar Afsana, Anant Kumar,
Maria de Lourdes Larrea and
Jennifer Hatfield

Objectives

- To review the importance of collaboration and partnership for global health
- To develop an understanding of the challenges and opportunities related to fostering global health collaborations and partnerships
- To foster an understanding of "partnership ethics" through examples

A) Introduction

Partnerships are central to global health. In this field, academics, practitioners and activists are constantly meeting and working with a variety of colleagues and patients from diverse communities. When approached with care, these relationships can be rich and beneficial (Royal Society 2011). Nurturing these relationships, and fostering strong and successful collaborations and partnerships, requires deliberate thought and action based on ethical conduct.

*We wish to acknowledge the contributions of Yves Talbot and Clément Habiyakere to the case studies in this chapter. We would also like to acknowledge the contributions of Aleida ter Kuile and Roberta Lloyd, whose hard work was essential to the success of the CCGHR's "Building Partnerships" project. Finally, we would like to acknowledge the generous contributions of the International Development Research Centre.

We define partnership as strategies that facilitate building, consolidating and sharing knowledge and expertise that contributes to promoting the goals of global health and building capacity (Canadian Coalition for Global Health Research (CCGHR) 2009). Partnerships can describe the way large-scale global health initiatives are funded, including public–private partnerships (e.g. Roll Back Malaria, Stop TB Partnership) and donor-country partnerships where governments of high-income countries (HICs) fund health programs in low- and middle-income countries (LMICs). Partnership may also refer to a way of working together with communities as an alternative to top-down initiatives. In the context of global health research, researchers from HICs and LMICs may collaborate to study complex challenges related to global health.

Much of the literature in this area pertains to research partnerships. Of equal importance are educational partnerships, which commonly take the form of joint degree programs between institutions in HICs and LMICs (Sewankambo 2011). These partnerships can be beneficial to each institution, and can help to fill a critical gap in training to support human resource capacity development in LMICs. Other types of partnership include those involving the actual delivery of clinical services and study placements, where a trainee is placed at another institution.

Understanding these different relationships is essential for ethical global health work. It helps in building trust between researchers, communities and institutions. This chapter provides examples of collaboration and partnership for global health, and of how principles such as social justice and solidarity (see Chapter 2) are realized through such relationships.

B) Benefits of partnerships

Partnerships are the result of a variety of motivations (Katz and Martin 1997) and benefits (Oldham 2005), which results in diverse impacts (Association of Universities and Colleges of Canada 2006).

Knowledge production

Research partnerships and collaborations may lead to the critical analysis of existing systems, the sharing of resources and the development of innovative interventions. According to Oldham (2005), scientists in LMICs often want to access the knowledge and expertise of their counterparts in HICs, in order to apply this knowledge to address local challenges. Importantly, knowledge sharing is certainly not a "one-way street." Partners from HICs and LMICs learn from one another, leading to broadened perspectives and new solutions to key challenges (Association of Universities and Colleges of Canada 2006). Researchers in HICs have a significant amount to learn from their colleagues in LMICs, for example about topics such as the control of diseases such as HIV/AIDS, malaria and TB and how to effectively use research findings to influence policymakers. For example in Cameroon, researchers have used policy briefs and stakeholder engagement to promote access to artemisinin-based combination therapies for malaria (Ongolo-Zogo and Bonono 2010).

Capacity development

Partnerships lead to strengthened capacity among individuals, institutions and systems in both HICs and in LMICs (Association of Universities and Colleges of Canada 2006; Bradley 2007). Strong, equitable and mutually beneficial research partnerships can lead to better health and health system outcomes (Bradley 2007). Again, researchers from HICs learn as much, if not more, from their LMIC colleagues, including increased knowledge of different cultural contexts and the adaptation of methodologies to various research contexts (Bradley 2007).

Access to resources

Access to both scientific (laboratories, equipment) and financial (grant money, institutional research budgets) resources is a benefit of collaboration (Oldham 2005). For example, research funding by organizations such as Canada's International Development Research Centre (IDRC) and the Swedish International Development Agency (SIDA) specifically promote collaboration as a key outcome of research initiatives.

Policy influence

Research partnerships between HICs and LMICs may often lead to new perspectives that inform or influence policy and subsequently address health challenges (Oldham 2005; Association of Universities and Colleges of Canada 2006).

C) Challenges of partnerships

Unequal access to resources

The reality of the disparity between LMICs and HICs is a major challenge to partnerships and a threat to equitable collaboration. This includes disparities in access to information (e.g. scientific literature), training and funding opportunities, international conferences and opportunities to publish. This is compounded by the dominance of languages such as English or French over local languages, and the dominance of Western knowledge and methods over local knowledge and methods (see Chapter 6). Bradley (2007) states that: "asymmetry between partners remains the principal obstacle to productive research collaboration" (*ibid.*: 2). Also detrimental, she states, is the "disproportionate influence of Northern partners in project administration and budget management" (*ibid.*). Similarly, Forti (2005) identifies inequalities in access to information and publishing opportunities as a major barrier to equity in partnerships. It is important to note that poor infrastructure and inefficient systems in LMICs may also be considered challenges for people from HICs working in LMICs. This may also be seen as a result of unequal access to resources, and requires long-term solutions.

Priority setting

Many LMICs have weak national health research systems and limited local sources available for research funding. This means that initiatives are generally funded by foreign donors, who often control the project's priorities (Forti 2005). Costello and Zumla (2000) state that: "[f]oreign domination in setting research priorities and project management may have negative consequences which outweigh the apparent benefits of the research findings" (Costello and Zumla 2000: 827).Therefore a lack of control of the research agenda by partners from LMICs might result in an imbalance of benefits in the favour of partners from HICs (Forti 2005; Oldham 2005.)

Exploitation

All too often, a pattern is seen whereby the academic partner from the LMIC will be employed as a data collector or research assistant, while their HIC counterpart takes on a leadership position (Oldham 2005). Partners from HICs may also fail to ensure that results from research are properly owned and controlled by local stakeholders. This, in turn, may lead to the research partnership being of great benefit to partners from HICs, while in fact being detrimental to their partners in LMICs. This may diminish the positive potential of the partnership to develop capacity, as described above. In order to avoid the exploitation of colleagues from LMICs, investment in long-term capacity development is needed to "level the playing field" and to balance power. In other words, where benefits exist as outlined above, risks are also present if partnerships are not properly designed and conducted.

Such challenges are reflective of the '10/90 Gap', where only 10 per cent of research funding is directed to health challenges that 90 per cent of the world's populations face (Commission on Health Research for Development 1990). Research funding is heavily weighted in favour of HICs, causing challenges to equity in health research. This can be seen throughout global health policy and practice.

D) Principles for conducting partnerships

The stated goal of global health partnerships is often the reduction of disparities in health outcomes. Hence, it is essential that institutional and organizational arrangements do not replicate the power differentials that are at the root of such disparities. Partnership ethics are guiding principles for the ways in which global health partnerships – in the fields of research, public health, medical practice and development projects – are conducted. Committing to partnership ethics is a commitment to ensure partnerships are enriching for all parties, in a way that brings no harm, supports mutual capacity development, and has an impact on health equity. Partnership ethics are based in a normative recognition of the need for equity in the way in which global health collaboration is carried out. It is useful to complement these normative principles with mechanisms that support equitable partnership practice. Engaging in equitable global health research partnerships requires deliberate and thoughtful input from all parties.

As Zarowsky (2011) states, it requires of collaborators "…listening, responsiveness, flexibility, willingness and capacity to follow as well as lead" (Zarowsky 2011: 1).

A number of principles for health research partnerships were advanced as a response to the flawed nature of many global health research partnerships. In its 1998 document *Guidelines for Research in Partnership with Developing Countries* (KFPE 1998), the Swiss Commission for Research Partnership with Developing Countries advanced eleven principles for health research partnerships*. These principles were developed to address the need for global research capacity to address critical world issues. The KFPE asserts that research partnerships are an effective way of improving LMICs' capacity to do effective and essential research, thus increasing the potential of finding solutions to major global challenges (*ibid.*). They suggested the following eleven partnership principles:

- Decide on the objectives
- Build up mutual trust
- Share information; develop networks
- Share responsibility
- Create transparency
- Monitor and evaluate the collaboration
- Disseminate the results
- Apply the results
- Share profits equitably
- Increase research capacity
- Build on the achievements

In 1999, the Netherlands Development Assistance Research Council (RAWOO) held an expert meeting on research partnership building, hosted by the Kerala Research Programme on Local Level Development (KRPLLD/IDS) at the Centre for Development Studies in Trivandrum, India. The meeting sought to generate discussion between actors from HICs and LMICs on a central question: "…is the current practice of North–South cooperation satisfactory to all concerned…?" (RAWOO 2001: 8). They defined "research cooperation" broadly as referring to collaboration that takes place between HICs and LMICs with a mandate for development. Six colleagues from LMICs made presentations about their experiences. The meeting resulted in the call for efforts on behalf of researchers in LMICs and HICs to work together to achieve the goal of "fruitful partnerships," and the recognition that constant effort is required so that "the effects of asymmetry…be neutralized." In the report, three guidelines for fruitful partnerships were advanced (*ibid.*: 29–30):

- Strengthening the capacity for conducting socially relevant research should be a specific aim of the partnership
- The Northern partner should be prepared to relinquish control and to accept considerable autonomy on the part of the Southern partner

---

*The KFPE revised the 11 principles in 2012. The revised principles can be accessed at: http://kfpe.ch/11_Principles/

- A broad-based consultative process, however painstaking and time-consuming it may be, should precede any programme

The report also calls for a paradigm shift in research, so that the "culture of the science system" better acknowledges socially relevant research, thus opening new channels for collaborative research (*ibid.*).

In 2000, Costello and Zumla advanced four broad principles for a partnership model to improve the practice of research in LMICs. They based their principles on a criticism of the practice of "annexed research" whereby researchers from HICs create research sites that are managed by expatriate staff, and often employ local people at inflated salaries. They argued that these "annexed" sites are damaging in that they attract local researchers away from national institutions and rarely involve sufficient local ownership to lead effective or appropriate policy influence (Costello and Zumla 2000). The principles are:

- Mutual trust and shared decision-making
- National ownership
- Emphasis on getting research findings into policy
- Development of national research capacity

There is a need to unpack the challenges of partnerships. These frameworks contain gaps, most notably the lack of Southern perspective on partnerships. The majority of what has been written about partnerships has been generated by academics or institutions from HICs. Similarly, much of what has been written about the benefits and challenges of global health research partnerships was also written in HICs and much of the discussion has occurred at the macro level. While important, there is little discussion of how the values can be put into action and into "real life" situations. While the Swiss, RAWOO and Costello and Zumla (2000) principles all capture key elements of what is needed to improve global health research partnerships, they do not give direction about what actions must be taken to achieve these goals. The Swiss principles do provide practical examples and checklists for each; Costello and Zumla (2000) also provide a checklist to accompany their principles. These checklists may be effective, but more direction is required to allow all partners to make use of them. Finally, the principles that each checklist advance are relevant primarily at the beginning of research partnerships. More guidance is needed to allow for such principles to be maintained throughout the duration of a partnership.

Box 9.1 Eliciting the "southern voice" in building effective and sustainable partnerships

The Canadian Coalition for Global Health Research (CCGHR or "the Coalition") is a non-governmental organization with the goal to "promote better and more equitable health worldwide through the production and use of knowledge" (CCGHR 2011). With the support of the IDRC, the Coalition was able to implement the Building Partnerships (BP) project. Consultations took place with researchers, decision-makers, funders, representatives of civil society organizations, and students in three regions: South Asia (Dhaka, Bangladesh), the Andean region of South America (Quito, Ecuador), and English-speaking Africa (Addis Ababa, Ethiopia).

The key finding was the reality of persistent inequity in the way health research partnerships are conducted and managed. Participants across the three regions spoke of negative partnership experiences in which Southern partners had been treated exploitatively and with disrespect, and where the partnership was exclusively beneficial to the most resourced partner – in particular, but not exclusively, partners from HICs. These inequities were felt not only between researchers or research institutions, but also between researchers and funders of research. During the African regional consultation in 2009, participants critiqued the "briefcase model" of health research partnerships, a model that many had experienced in practice. This involved researchers from the North arriving to "fill their briefcases" with data to take back to their home country or institution. Within this model, capable researchers from the South were often relegated to the tasks of data collection, and were unacknowledged in subsequent dissemination of findings such as papers and conference presentations.

Inequity often persists due to an unequal balance of resources, as funds and technology are often controlled by Northern institutions. There is also a lack of discussion and formal agreement about the terms of the partnership and a failure to articulate clearly the interests, benefits and contributions of each partner. The absence of formal agreements often leads to a lack of leverage for negotiation for the less resourced partners.

A key resource that emerged from this project is the Partnership Assessment Tool (PAT), developed by academics from LMICs, which guides participants throughout the stages of partnership development (available at www.ccghr.ca).

Case study 9.1

Capacity development for primary health care management: a Canada–Brazil partnership

The University of Toronto's Department of Family and Community Medicine (DFCM) has worked in partnership with colleagues and institutions in Brazil for over a decade to increase primary health care capacity in the country. In 2007, the DFCM responded to a request by the Brazilian Ministry of Health to develop the Primary Health Care Management (AGAP) project, to strengthen capacity in primary health care while promoting gender and racial equality. The project took place in four states and involved forty-one projects in each state. The program integrated capacity development in four areas – care, management, training and communication – and involved managers, clients and their families from the communities served. The project led to improved capacity and increased quality of care in previously underserved disease areas such as tuberculosis and leprosy.

Several challenges arose during the AGAP project. Cultural difference was an important factor: the bureaucratic culture of the Canadian funding environment was unfamiliar to many of the Brazilian colleagues, requiring careful translation of expectations between teams to ensure all requirements were met. Similarly, linguistic differences between Canadian and Brazilian colleagues had to be navigated. This was mitigated by translating lectures by Canadian partners into Portuguese so that they could be re-used for future training sessions.

Building trust over time was essential, as was the initiation by the Brazilian side. The AGAP project was mutually beneficial in that Canadian and Brazilian teams learned from each other. Brazil has carried out the largest primary health care reform in the world, and this was of great interest to Canadians working in the primary health care field in Canada. Brazilian colleagues were able to learn from Canadians about approaches to specific health challenges such as mental health.

Case study 9.2

Global health partnership in Zambia

The Zambia Forum for Health Research (ZAMFOHR) is a non-governmental organization specializing in knowledge translation. Its goal is to: "improve the health quality of Zambians by ensuring that health research evidence forms the basis for the policy and practice that drives the healthcare system" (ZAMFOHR n.d.). Master's of Public Health students attending Simon Fraser University have worked within ZAMFOHR to conduct locally relevant research, often with the mentorship of faculty at the University of Zambia. This has facilitated access to key informants and ensured that all research is done within the context of ZAMFOHR's strategic initiatives. Partnerships have been mutually beneficial for students and Zambian faculty.

Training and retention of health professionals is a challenge faced by many LMICs. The Catholic University of Health and Allied Sciences-Bugando (CUHAS-Bugando) is one of two medical universities certified to train physicians outside Tanzania's capital. The Department of Community Medicine had attempted to develop a Master of Public Health (MPH) program for several years, but capacity and resource challenges held up progress. Based on a history of previous collaboration, the leadership of CUHAS-Bugando invited the University of Calgary to help in developing the MPH Program. Representatives from both universities collaborated on the development of a curriculum, with University of Calgary faculty playing a key role in curriculum delivery through the first years of the program. Simultaneously, local staff were to be trained, with responsibility for teaching being passed on to CUHAS-Bugando staff.

During 2010–11, twenty University of Calgary faculty travelled to Tanzania to collaborate on the first year of the MPH program. The first eight students graduated in November 2011, with the rest of the inaugural class expected to graduate in early 2012. The second year is now under way, and two MPH graduates have been hired by CUHAS-Bugando to begin building long-term capacity.

Challenges faced along the way included concerns by University of Calgary faculty about receiving support in terms of safety, transportation and orientation while visiting Tanzania. CUHAS-Bugando representatives shared their concerns about commitment and the sustainability of the partnership. Also of major concern to both parties was the concept of capacity building. The University of Calgary's goal was to build the capacity of faculty to engage in educational experiences and research in resource-constrained settings. They wanted to learn from Tanzanian colleagues how public health challenges were managed in a country that faced urban and rural divides, indigenous populations that experience worse health outcomes and significant human resource challenges. The Tanzanian partners were very interested in building their capacity to run a high-quality nationally recognized MPH.

The approach taken to negotiating the partnerships and discussing these concerns was crucial to the success of this partnership. The partners made use of the PAT, drawing on it to guide frank and open discussions through the "inception phase" of the partnership. Using the PAT created a safe environment in which both parties could be open about their motivations and interests.

Case study 9.4

Building capacity and promoting community-based impact: the Ecuador Eco-Health Initiative

The University of British Columbia; the National Institute of Hygiene, Epidemiology and Microbiology in Cuba; and Mexico's National Institute of Public Health have partnered with universities in Ecuador on the Ecuador Eco-Health Initiative, which seeks to build a community of practice to support environmental health in Ecuador.

Since it began in 2004, its Master's program, which takes a participatory action approach, has led to community-based impact that ranges from the development of dengue prevention programs to the identification and prevention of lead poisoning in the artisanal community of San Jose de Balzay. Its PhD program in Society, Environment and Health is a partnership between the University of British Columbia, the University Andina Simon Bolívar, FIOCRUZ in Brazil and the Andean Health organization. This program benefits students from all Andean countries. The project has also been successful in building capacity among Ecuadoran master's and doctoral graduates, which enables them to remain, and to build careers, in the Andean region (Speigel et al. 2011). This means the impact of this partnership will be felt long after students have graduated and will be of lasting benefit for the region.

E) Conclusion

Ethics and equity must be at the heart of partnerships in order for them to be successful. Partnering is not just a way in which to get things done – it is about people and relationships, and therefore must be approached with care, thought and consideration. Students engaging in partnerships must also recognize the bigger picture of global health, grounded in the desire to improve health outcomes and health equity on a global scale. Successful partnerships depend on ethical conduct. Not only that, successful partnerships are also more likely to lead to results that influence health policy, practice and outcomes to have a real impact. In the course of their careers, students might be faced with situations in which they recognize unethical conduct in partnerships.

This chapter draws on the experiences of its authors. Some key additional recommendations are as follows.

- Before entering into a partnership or collaboration, consider motivations. Ask yourself if the relationship will benefit you specifically, or if it will be mutually beneficial. Ask yourself if you are perpetuating the "briefcase model" or are entering into a true collaboration. Ask whether what you are doing will add value (for example through knowledge production) on a broader scale.

- Be aware that learning is a two-way street. Ask yourself what you can learn from your colleagues and the communities with whom you are working. Ask yourself what you can learn from your patients or clients. Ask yourself what they can learn from you.
- Check in frequently on the health of your partnership – is everyone involved happy, learning and able to work to their full capacity? If a problem arises, are you able to discuss it in an open and honest way?

References

Association of Universities and Colleges of Canada (2006) *Highlighting the Impacts of North–South Research Collaboration among Canadian and Southern Higher Education Partners*. Ottawa: Association of Universities and Colleges of Canada.

Bradley, M. (2007) *North–South Research Partnerships: Challenges, Responses and Trends; a Literature Review and Annotated Bibliography*. Canadian Partnerships Working Paper #1. Ottawa: International Development Research Centre.

CCGHR (2009) *Partnership Assessment Tool*. Ottawa: Canadian Coalition for Global Health Research. www.ccghr.ca/Resources/Documents/Resources/PAT_Interactive_e.pdf

— (2011) *About Us*. www.ccghr.ca/about_us

Commission on Health Research for Development (1990) *Health Research: Essential Link to Equity in Development*. New York: Oxford University Press.

Costello, A. and Zumla, A. (2000) 'Moving to research partnerships in developing countries', *British Medical Journal*, 321: 827–29.

Forti, S. (2005) *Building Partnerships for Research in Global Health: Analytical Framework*. Ottawa: Canadian Coalition for Global Health Research.

Katz, J.S. and Martin, B.R. (1997) 'What is research collaboration?', *Research Policy*, 26(1): 1–18.

KFPE (1998) *Guidelines for Research in Partnership with Developing Countries: 11 Principles*. Swiss Commission for Research Partnership with Developing Countries. www.kfpe.ch/key_activities/publications/guidelines/guidelines_e.php

Oldham, G. (2005) *International Scientific Collaboration: A Quick Guide*. Science and Development Network. www.scidev.net/en/policy-briefs/international-scientific-collaboration-a-quick-gui.html

Ongolo-Zogo, P. and Bonono, R.-C. (2010) 'Policy brief on improving access to artemisinin-based combination therapies for malaria in Cameroon', *International Journal of Technology Assessment in Health Care*, 26: 237–41.

RAWOO (2001) *North–South Research Partnerships: Issues and Challenges. Trivandrum Expert Meeting Report, 1999*. The Hague: RAWOO.

Royal Society (2011) *Knowledge, Networks and Nations: Global Scientific Collaboration in the 21st Century*, RS Policy Document 03/11. London: The Royal Society.

Sewankambo, N. (2011) 'The value and challenges of institutional partnerships in global health: a view from the South', in: *Building Institutions Through Equitable Partnerships in Global Health Conference*, Royal College of Physicians, London, 14–15 April. www.rcplondon.ac.uk/policy/reducing-health-harms/global-health/global-partnerships-2011

Speigel, J. et al. (2011) 'Establishing a community of practice of researchers, practitioners, policy-makers and communities to sustainably manage environmental health risks in Ecuador', *BMC International Health and Human Rights*, 11(Suppl. 2).

ZAMFOHR (n.d.) *About ZAMFOHR*. Lusaka: Zambia Forum for Health Research. www.zamfohr.org/aboutus.html

Zarowsky, C. (2011) 'Global health research, partnership, and equity: no more business-as-usual', *BMC International Health and Human Rights*, 11(Suppl. 2).

10 | Perspectives on global health from the South

Ana Sanchez and Victor A. López

Objectives

- To discuss reasons for the under-representation in the literature on global health from Southern authors based in the South, despite collaboration with Northern partners
- To consider guidelines and recommendations for ethical conduct being developed for students, researchers and countries in the North collaborating with LMICs

A) Introduction

The existing body of literature on global health – its evolving definitions, scope and, very importantly, the values and competencies required for ethical practice – reveals a troubling imbalance: there is little contribution from Southern authors based in the South. This under-representation is even more striking when considering the enormous growth in global health activity, particularly the hosting of Northern partners as part of the myriad of research and training opportunities taking place in low- and middle-income countries (LMICs). Undoubtedly such opportunities are beneficial for the arriving guests (Crump and Sugarman 2008; Fennell 2009; Plugge and Cole 2011), but are they beneficial to the hosts? Laabes et al. (2011) suggest that while some African schools receive much needed funding from an ever-increasing number of European and American graduate programs, these collaborations often perpetuate "post-colonial syndrome," a legacy of reckless, exploitative and unequal interactions (Laabes et al. 2011). Conversely, Glew (2008) argues that not all Western investigators are necessarily cultural imperialists, and prefers to believe his American students and colleagues when they express noble motives for undertaking research or studies in Africa (Glew 2008). An examination of the impact of study-abroad students in Chilean institutions and society concludes that these opportunities can contribute greatly to world peace through a better understanding of different values and cultures in both the sojourner and the host (Stephenson 1999).

B) Guidelines for international collaborations

The growing consensus is, however, that international training experiences may be a substantial burden on already resource-constrained hosts (Redwood-Campbell et al. 2011). Moreover, recognizing that considerably less attention has been given to the ethics of global health training than to global health research, the Working Group on Ethics Guidelines for Global Health Training (WEIGHT) guidelines have been proposed. These suggest best practices for Northern students, teachers, donors and institutions engaged in global health training experiences in LMICs (Crump and Sugarman 2010). In addition to addressing ethical conflicts emerging from international service learning programs, other authors have expanded the scope of ethical conduct and incorporated recommendations related to project sustainability and community involvement (Reisch 2011). In particular, the concept of capacity-building in the South has evolved from simply a desirable outcome to a vital measure of the ethical value of undertaking of these partnerships (Ijsselmuiden et al. 2010; Bates et al. 2011).

Similar to the challenges surrounding training activities, the global health enterprise at large can also be plagued by ethical concerns (Ijsselmuiden et al. 2010) and can perpetuate the very inequities it is seeking to address (Costello and Zumla 2000). Acknowledging that North–South research collaboration is essential for the advancement of science and society, in 2008 a Working Group on International Research Collaborations (I-Group) was formed in the United States to look systematically at international research collaborations. As part of its activities, a Workshop on Examining Core Elements of International Collaboration was held in July 2010. The report from the workshop is rich in case studies and suggestions, concluding that there is a need to put together a "primer or guide that would outline the necessary steps in forming and undertaking various types of collaboration," and inherently one that would ascertain possible pitfalls of such collaborations, as well as provide insight for understanding and managing potential risks that may arise from such endeavors (Sauer and Arrison 2011) (see also Chapter 9). Indeed, as the global health field continues to expand, an additional need for global health diplomacy expertise has begun to emerge (Kickbusch et al. 2007).

Notwithstanding these efforts, and the fact that existing or future guidelines for best practices on global health training and research can be interpreted and adapted by recipient LMICs, the voices from the South are yet to be heard in the same explicit mode and in international spaces. The manner and mechanisms in which training and research partnerships are agreed upon and implemented in the South for the most part go unrecorded. There are a few exceptions, however, documenting North–South research cooperation, although none explicitly suggests guidelines for equitable cooperation.

A recent article analyzing four successful projects between African countries and the Liverpool School of Tropical Medicine identifies criteria for sustainable capacity-building and emphasizes the importance of promoting local ownership from the onset (Bates et al. 2011). An additional example is an article recounting the experience of scientific cooperation between Zimbabwe and Denmark, which demonstrates a long-standing relationship that was able to endure cultural and political differences

(Chandiwana and Ornbjerg 2003). The authors propose "Most institutions in developing countries, particularly those in Africa, are too weak to participate effectively in joint research programs with institutions in industrialized countries" (*ibid.*: 293). They also conclude that autonomy and capacity-building, including research leadership, are crucial for an effective and sustainable role in research productivity and North–South as well as South–South cooperation (Chandiwana and Ornbjerg 2003).

Publications from developing countries in Latin America that effectively engage in global health activities with countries from the North are even more difficult to find in the literature. An exception to this is a recent paper from Central America that illustrates the development of scientific capacity over a period of more than twenty years with the assistance of the Swedish International Development Cooperation Agency (Moreno et al. 2011). In this case, the ultimate objective of the cooperation program was improving the sustainability of scientific research in the region through the creation of NeTropica, a not-for-profit organization with the mandate of funding local research and sustaining a network for knowledge exchange. NeTropica has operated successfully for ten years; unfortunately, its future is uncertain unless it can secure ongoing funding from local and international partners (Moreno et al. 2011).

These examples provide hope that egalitarian partnerships may be more common than previously thought. On the other hand, they may illustrate a publication bias whereby success stories may be more amenable to report (Corbin et al. 2011). By the same token, they may exemplify situations of official bilateral agreements that were initiated due to the needs of the Southern partner and may not be reflective of smaller-scale interactions between institutions and/or academics. Of the latter, the perception exists that training needs are fulfilled and research interests prioritized to the detriment (sometimes overt but more often subtle) of the hosting developing country, but the paucity of published work makes it difficult to ascertain its validity and to offer recommendations on how to promote more equitable collaborations.

In the absence of substantial written evidence, the question may arise: are researchers and institutions based in resource-constrained countries interested in producing guidelines for partnership setting with the North? The international literature is scarce on this issue, but there is reason to believe such interest exists. A good example of these emerging voices is an article by Adamson Muula from Malawi, who asks researchers to refrain from issuing "condescending, paternalistic and offensive" descriptions of his country, and suggests ethical guidelines for taking photographs of peoples and places (Muula 2010).

A second, even more important question also remains: do Southerners in global health alliances feel empowered enough to believe that their guidelines – if produced – will be taken seriously when negotiating agreements? When searching for answers, the contextual aspects of these questions need to be kept in mind. Facing serious economic and social challenges, the prioritization of research may not be at the top of LMIC governments' agendas.

To bring life to this abstract discussion, the following three case studies are offered to exemplify views on global health from the South, specifically in terms of hosting students from the North (Case 10.1), experiences of individual research collaboration (Case 10.2) and authorship (Case 10.3).

Case study 10.1

Hosting students from the North

Every year, hundreds of undergraduate and graduate students from the North travel to Guatemala and Honduras to take part in different training initiatives in global health, including research and service activities.

The visiting students are generally well received and usually are provided with access to procedures and experiences that are not usual in their home countries. In most cases, foreign students are given privileges and preferences that are not afforded to local students. Additionally, receiving visitors entails a variety of time-consuming duties for the host institutions and personnel, including supervision, guidance, tutoring and socializing. Even when universities from the North are appreciative of these efforts, they are commonly performed in a "collaborative" way without economic compensation or academic recognition for the hosts. Similarly, the actual and direct benefits for the country and the population are not always clear. Hosting student placements can be unfair to countries in the South, even when it seeks to address issues such as inequity and social injustice.

Case study 10.2

North–South collaborations may start well, but their fate is sometimes uncertain

"We have always wanted to help find a solution for a health condition affecting livestock and people in our country, so we approached a group of researchers from a developed country that had produced and was testing a treatment for the disease in animals. They were happy to entertain our ideas and accepted our country as a research site. With our own funding, we tested the treatment using a very expensive, rigorous and ethical experimental protocol. The one-year trial was a success and we were interested in doing a larger study. We sent samples to the foreign researchers' lab for some additional testing, but a year passed without feedback. Every so often we would ask for results, but our emails went unanswered. One day we were finally told that our findings didn't show anything new as they already had proof of the treatment's efficacy; they were also busy testing the treatment at a larger scale elsewhere so could not continue working with us. This was extremely disappointing and made us regret having spent our resources and time on this study. Finally, in an attempt to rescue something, we asked if at least we could publish the results, but they said that the study didn't prove anything new and was now too old to be published. That was the last time we heard from them." (Source: a biomedical researcher from the South.)

Even though proficient researchers in less developed countries are indeed capable of initiating collaboration with researchers in the North, an equitable and lasting partnership can develop only when both parties perceive the association as mutually beneficial and synergizing. There is also a need to establish a written agreement that explicitly outlines each partner's expectations and obligations at the outset.

Case study 10.3

Global health research and equitable authorship

At the end of a collaborative project with Northern partners, a group of researchers and practitioners from the South expressed the tensions arising when negotiating the dissemination strategy. For the Northern side of the team, however, the most pressing issue was to publish in English language peer-reviewed journals, as within their context this kind of output is highly valued and an indication of success. For the Southern colleagues, the priority was to produce reports and presentations to engage local decision-makers and the communities where research participants were recruited. They asserted that the granting agency's project evaluation framework did not fully consider the realities and priorities of developing countries. Further, the Southern researchers stated that, albeit desirable, publications were not necessarily the ultimate research output: many collaborative projects seek to build capacity (strengthen processes, transfer technology, form mentors, instill leadership) and, although their achievements can, and perhaps should, be counted and recounted, the individual, institutional and societal transformations stemming from them are far better indicators of success than a handful of publications. They also emphasized that, more often than not, LMICs' decision-makers and research-users are either unaware of such publications, have no access to them, or simply cannot understand the jargon (and sometimes the language) in which they are written.

This underscores the need for a mutual understanding with regard to the value, weight and relevance of research publications. Few in the North would negate the importance and appropriateness of research dissemination in LMIC. However, what is perhaps needed is an evolution of the "peer-review" concept and an expansion of project evaluation criteria that bestow equal merit on a variety of forms and channels that global health researchers must utilize for knowledge sharing.

C) Recommendations

It is imperative that scientific collaboration between researchers, institutions and countries – whether for training, research, or both – operates under the guiding principles of reciprocity, solidarity and social justice. This is particularly important where one of the partners may be more vulnerable due to historic, economic or political reasons. To this extent, it is commendable that guidelines and recommendations for ethical conduct are being developed for students, researchers and countries in the North. Of equal importance, LMIC stakeholders should endeavor to develop similar regulations based on their own insights and perspectives, thus bringing their essential voices to the dynamic conversation about the ethics of global health – one that continues to be dominated by Northern voices.

References

Bates, I., Taegtmeyer, M., Squire, S.B., Ansong, D., Nhlema-Simwaka, B., Baba, A. and Theobald, S. (2011) 'Indicators of sustainable capacity building for health research: analysis of four African case studies', *Health Research Policy and Systems*, 9: 14.

Chandiwana, S. and Ornbjerg, N. (2003) 'Review of North–South and South–South cooperation and conditions necessary to sustain research capability in developing countries', *Journal of Health, Population, and Nutrition*, 21: 288–97.

Corbin, J.H., Mittelmark, M.B. and Lie, G.T. (2011) 'Mapping synergy and antagony in North–South partnerships for health: a case study of the Tanzanian women's NGO KIWAKKUKI', *Health Promotion International*, 15 December.

Costello, A. and Zumla, A. (2000) 'Moving to research partnerships in developing countries', *British Medical Journal*, 321: 827–29.

Crump, J.A. and Sugarman, J. (2008) 'Ethical considerations for short-term experiences by trainees in global health', *JAMA*, 300: 1456–58.

— (2010) 'Ethics and best practice guidelines for training experiences in global health', *American Journal of Tropical Medicine and Hygiene*, 83: 1178–82.

Fennell, R. (2009) 'The impact of an international health study abroad program on university students from the United States', *Global Health Promotion*, 16: 17–23.

Glew, R.H. (2008) 'Promoting collaborations between biomedical scholars in the U.S. and sub-Saharan Africa', *Experimental Biogy and Medicine (Maywood)*, 233: 277–85.

Ijsselmuiden, C.B., Kass, N.E., Sewankambo, K.N. and Lavery, J.V. (2010) 'Evolving values in ethics and global health research', *Global Public Health*, 5: 154–63.

Kickbusch, I., Novotny, T.E., Drager, N., Silberschmidt, G. and Alcazar, S. (2007) 'Global health diplomacy: training across disciplines', *Bulletin of the World Health Organization*, 85: 971–73.

Laabes, E.P., Desai, R., Zawedde, S.M. and Glew, R.H. (2011) 'How much longer will Africa have to depend on western nations for support of its capacity-building efforts for biomedical research?', *Tropical Medicine & International Health*, 16: 258–62.

Moreno, E., Gutierrez, J.M. and Chaves-Olarte, E. (2011) 'The struggle of neglected scientific groups: ten years of NeTropica efforts to promote research in tropical diseases in Central America', *PLoS Neglected Tropical Diseases*, 5: e1055.

Muula, A.S. (2010) 'We are not just a "tiny, landlocked, impoverished sub-Saharan country with HIV burden"', *Croatian Medical Journal*, 51: 560–62.

Plugge, E. and Cole, D. (2011) 'Oxford graduates' perceptions of a global health master's degree: a case study', *Human Resources for Health*, 9: 26.

Redwood-Campbell, L., Pakes, B., Rouleau, K., Macdonald, C.J., Arya, N., Purkey, E., Schultz, K., Dhatt, R., Wilson, B., Hadi, A. and Pottie, K. (2011) 'Developing a curriculum framework for global health in family medicine: emerging principles, competencies, and educational approaches', *BMC Medical Education*, 11: 46.

Reisch, R.A. (2011) 'International service learning programs: ethical issues and recommendations', *Developing World Bioethics*, 11: 93–98.

Sauer, S. and Arrison, T. (2011) *Examining Core Elements of International Research Collaboration: Summary of a Workshop*. Washington, DC: National Academies Press.

Stephenson, S. (1999) 'Study abroad as a transformational experience and its effect upon study abroad students and host nationals in Santiago, Chile', *Frontiers: The Interdisciplinary Journal of Study Abroad*, 5: 1–38.

11

The political context of global health and advocacy

Nathan Ford

Objectives

- To offer an overview of global health advocacy
- To introduce a framework for global health advocacy that draws on policy analysis

A) Introduction

The practice of health advocacy has existed for hundreds of years. Rudolf Virchow's (1840) often-cited claim that "Medicine is a social science, and politics is nothing else but medicine on a large scale" (cited in Sigerist 1941: 93) may be seen as recognition of intensive health activism taking place at that time. In the United Kingdom, for example, campaigning by pressure groups to promote the sanitary reform brought about the 1848 Public Health Act (Berridge 2007).

Global health advocacy – which could be defined as people in one part of the world advocating for the improved health of people in another part of the world – also has a long history. Recent advocacy efforts to draw attention to the lack of drug development for neglected tropical diseases of the developing world (Barry 2003) are the latest in a 100-year-long struggle to control these diseases (Janssens et al. 1992).

In a world driven by humanitarian concerns alone, funding would be prioritized according to medical and public health need, with particular attention to factors such as marginalization and discrimination that deliberately promote poor health among certain groups, or exclude them from accessing care. Unfortunately, such a global health utopia does not exist. In reality, national interests play a substantial role in donors' decisions to respond to major health challenges. Just as colonial interests drove the United Kingdom's tropical disease research in the first half of the twentieth century (see Chapter 1), more recent international efforts to fight diseases such as HIV, tuberculosis and malaria have, in part, been driven by diplomacy and national security considerations (Feldbaum et al. 2010). This can have mixed or even contradictory consequences. For example, national security concerns formed part of the US government's decisions to invest in global funding for HIV (Feldbaum et al. 2006), resulting in the largest international funding effort against a single disease (Ford et al. 2011). At the same time, however, domestic trade interests led the US government to lobby for trade rules that protected the patents of pharmaceutical companies and limited access to the most affordable treatments for HIV.

This chapter provides an overview of global health advocacy, introducing the reader to a useful framework that draws on policy analysis. Advocacy efforts to increase access to HIV treatment will be illustrated as a key example.

B) A framework for global health advocacy

There are a number of features common to successful global health advocacy campaigns. The first step is defining the problem, which in general should be political in nature – that is to say, amenable to a political solution. For example, if a medicine is expensive because the manufacturing process is complex and labour-intensive, then advocacy will be of little use. However, if a medicine is known to be cheap to make, but is sold at a very high price, then public pressure may be effective in reducing the price. Such public pressure creates political tension that can force governments to intervene, for example by negotiating discounts from pharmaceutical companies, or seeking generic alternatives to more expensive patented drugs. Next, evidence needs to be gathered to support the case. In the era of evidence-based health care, policy makers will usually require data to substantiate the importance of a particular health problem. Then, for advocacy to be successful, a clear policy solution needs to be proposed. At the same time, allies need to be identified to help support the case that the issue of concern is not a marginal one, but matters to a range of stakeholders. Opportunities to promote the solution will arise, and these need to be seized. Finally, if successful, advocates should be ready to play a supportive role in implementation of the solution.

In reality, policy change does not occur in a linear fashion, and advocacy rarely takes such a stepwise approach. According to health policy theory, opportunities to change policy ("policy windows") arise only when three separate and independently evolving streams – problems, policies and politics – converge. Advocacy efforts aim to influence these three different streams, and need to evolve rapidly in response to opening and closing of policy windows (Kingdon 1984).

Nevertheless, a stepwise framework is useful for outlining distinct stages in an advocacy campaign. In this chapter, the framework is used to describe advocacy efforts to improve access to treatment for HIV in Africa.

Example: Access to treatment for people living with HIV in Africa

Defining the problem

The first step in any advocacy effort is to agree on the problem that needs to be overcome. There are an overwhelming number of examples of inequalities in health care around the world, and reasonable people can hold different or even opposing views about which problem should take priority.

Medicines to treat HIV have been available since the first antiretroviral drug, zidovudine, was marketed in 1987. But it was only with the advent of triple therapy in 1996 that major gains were made in long-term survival for people living with HIV (Ford et al. 2011). For decades, the greatest burden of HIV has been in Africa. In 2001, some 20.3 million people were living with HIV in sub-Saharan Africa. According to more recent estimates, that figure is now 22.5 million (UNAIDS 2010). Initially, antiretroviral medicines were priced out of reach for the majority of people in need, costing more than $10,000 per patient/year in developing and developed countries alike, and there was considerable disagreement about whether the focus of attention should be on prevention or treatment. For example, researchers at the World Health Organization (WHO) concluded, on the basis of a review of cost-effectiveness data at the time, that prevention should take precedence over treatment in developing countries (Creese et al. 2002). Others argued that health systems in sub-Saharan Africa could not cope with the strain of providing treatment to millions of patients in need (McCoy et al. 2005). Concern was even expressed that adherence to treatment in Africa would be suboptimal (Attaran 2007).

Civil society groups, and in particular people living with HIV, played a central role in arguing the case that access to treatment had to become a major international political priority. Patient groups in Thailand, Brazil, South Africa, India, Kenya, Uganda and other high-burden countries formed alliances with health providers, NGOs and health groups in developed countries to argue the case that the cost of treatment was too high and must be reduced (Ford et al. 2011). The fact that life-saving treatment existed, but was not being made available to those in greatest need because of the high cost of the medicines, was considered unacceptable and a violation of human rights (see Chapter 4). The politicization of the problem came from the understanding that drug prices were not a reasonable reflection of the cost of researching, developing and manufacturing, but were artificially high and based on the profits sought by pharmaceutical companies.

Thus, while not universally accepted, there was sufficiently broad agreement among groups in both developed and developing countries that access to life-saving treatment needed to be improved, and this became an advocacy priority for much of the next decade.

Gathering the evidence

Advocacy for scale-up of antiretroviral therapy relied on at least three different types of data: epidemiological data, drug pricing data and treatment efficacy data.

Data describing the burden of HIV disease was essential to building the case that treatment was a priority. In 1999, the United Nations (UN) published epidemiological data that outlined the following points: there were an estimated 33.6 million HIV-infected individuals, 23.3 million of them living in Africa; in 1999, there were 5.6 million new infections, with the majority, 3.8 million, again in Africa; since the epidemic began, there have been 2.6 million AIDS-related deaths; and life expectancy in much of the continent dropped to forty-five years or less (UNAIDS 2000). These data, which are now published annually as part of the UNAIDS global HIV/AIDS epidemic update, formed the basis for advocacy and for expanded efforts to improve treatment and care for people living with HIV worldwide.

The availability of comparative drug-pricing data also proved critical to advocacy efforts. The fact that in early 2000 antiretroviral therapy was priced out of reach of those in need was recognized as a problem at the highest political levels. However, in the absence of data to demonstrate the inequalities in pricing of medicines around the world, the high price of drugs was not challenged. That pharmaceutical companies spent money on drug research and development, and that these companies needed to recoup their investments, was accepted as a fact. The collection and publication of pricing data for medicines to treat HIV and opportunistic infections helped to challenge this argument. In 2000, Médecins Sans Frontières (MSF) published data from countries in Asia, Africa and Latin America that showed a 100-fold variation in the price of fluconazole, a drug to treat AIDS-related meningitis (Perez-Casas et al. 2000). MSF, the WHO and other UN agencies also published pricing surveys for selected drugs used in the care of people living with HIV (UNICEF et al. 2000). Such data have been critical to ensure ongoing pressure on pharmaceutical companies to lower the price of antiretroviral medicines for developing countries, and have formed the basis of policy discussions towards greater flexibility in international law to allow countries to access the best available prices on the global pharmaceutical market (Hoen et al. 2011).

Finally, early treatment outcome data demonstrating the safety and efficacy of providing antiretroviral therapy in resource-limited settings helped convince international donors and national governments that the provision of antiretroviral therapy was a life-saving public health priority (Kasper et al. 2003).

Championing a solution

Up until 2000, the high cost of antiretroviral medicines excluded widespread access to treatment in Africa. Although there had been calls in the past for reducing the prices charged by pharmaceutical companies, these were by and large comfortably ignored (Altman 2006).

The potential for antiretroviral drugs to be manufactured at substantially lower prices was being explored by two middle-income countries with a high burden of people living with HIV – Brazil and Thailand (Ford et al. 2007). However, such initiatives were focused mainly on developing affordable medicines for their own populations, with no major ambition to produce medicines for export to other countries.

A major breakthrough came in 2001, when the Indian generics company Cipla announced that it could manufacture triple therapy for US$350 per person per year (Hoen et al. 2011). It rapidly became clear that the global patent rules that permitted or hindered the international movement of medicines, as determined by the World Trade Agreements, had a major influence over the ability of developing countries to be able to access generic drugs at the price being offered by the Indian manufacturers.

The availability of affordable generic antiretrovirals in India represented a solution that could help drive an advocacy strategy both to pressure other companies to lower the prices of their medicines and, at the same time, to encourage governments and intergovernmental agencies to support the export of Indian generic drugs to Africa.

Building alliances

In order to build the case that increased access to antiretroviral therapy should be a priority, expertise and experience from a range of fields was required. Intellectual property experts provided an analysis of the legal aspects of international and national laws that determined the possibility of overriding patents in order to manufacture and export generic medicines. Clinicians gave advice about which drugs were most urgently required and, through treating patients as soon as medicines were available, provided evidence that treating HIV in resource-limited settings was feasible. In order to address concerns about poor adherence and the risk of drug resistance, researchers gathered and synthesized data that showed that adherence to treatment in Africa was as good as, if not better than, adherence in North America (Mills et al. 2006). Health economists modelled data to show that treating HIV was cost-effective. NGOs launched public campaigns to challenge pharmaceutical patents and support access to medicines in trade laws. Pharmacists advised on the quality of generic versions of patent drugs. And, perhaps most importantly, the voices of patients themselves articulated the urgency of the need.

One of the landmark cases illustrating the strength of such collaborative efforts was a court case that took place in South Africa. Between 1997 and 2001, a consortium of thirty-nine pharmaceutical companies litigated against the government of South Africa, which at the time was trying to pass a Medicines Act that would allow for the import of medicines being sold at a lower price in neighbouring countries. At that time (and still today), South Africa was the country with the largest number of people living with HIV, estimated at around 5.6 million. A dedicated advocacy campaign was mounted against the court case, bringing together a coalition of lawyers, doctors, NGOs and local and international activist groups. A local activist group, the Treatment Action Campaign, challenged the court case on the grounds that it was a violation of the human right to health. MSF co-ordinated a petition that collected over 250,000 signatures. These and other actions led to such forceful international public pressure that the pharmaceutical industry was forced to drop the case (Forman 2008; Hoen et al. 2011).

Challenging the status quo

By definition, advocacy is confrontational because it involves, at least in the early stages, challenging the *status quo*. The proposal that the needs of patients in developing countries should be prioritized over the patents of pharmaceutical companies and that affordable generic medicines should be purchased in order to scale-up treatment was, in 2000, a radical idea that met with strong opposition from Western governments. The pharmaceutical industry tried to deflect attention, arguing that the price of medicines was not the most important issue, and that efforts should first address poverty rather than medical patents (GlaxoSmithKline 2011). UN officials who conducted investigations into pharmaceutical pricing policies were threatened, sometimes violently (Vidal 2001). Western governments, protecting the interests of their domestic pharmaceutical industries, threatened trade sanctions against developing countries that attempted to override medical patents (Wilson et al. 1999). The establishment of broad coalitions was essential to help overcome these pressures and provide political support to groups that may otherwise have been forced to abandon the cause.

Seizing opportunities

Opportunism has played an important part in furthering global advocacy to support access to affordable HIV medicines. The decision by the consortium of pharmaceutical industries to sue the South African government was an unplanned opportunity that turned into a public relations disaster for the pharmaceutical industry. The case was portrayed in the media as a "David and Goliath" battle that pitted the health of millions of poor Africans' health against the corporate wealth of billion-dollar drug companies (Hoen et al. 2011). The publicity around the case helped garner global public attention around an issue that was previously seen as a technical legal issue.

In late 2001, responding to a perceived threat of terrorism, the US government took steps to secure a stockpile of generic ciprofloxacin, the antibiotic to treat anthrax, because the patented drug was considered too expensive. The example was immediately seized upon as an instance of global health hypocrisy, given that the US government was, at the time, lobbying to protect industry interests and limit the ability of developing countries to access generic antiretroviral drugs. The publicity generated helped to garner support for the Ministerial Doha Declaration in 2001 that prioritized public health over patents in trade negotiations that were taking place at the time (Boseley 2001).

Building consensus

Advocacy will fail if everyone agrees on the problem but disagrees on the solution. Initially, while most health advocacy groups agreed that access to HIV medicines needed to be improved, there was some disagreement among advocacy groups about what solution should be defended. Should the public health safeguards that are written into trade law be defended, or should the laws be rewritten completely? Divergent views existed about what solution to push for. Some campaigners took the view that the current intellectual property system was flawed and should be scrapped altogether (Tickell 2001). Others considered this to be a high-risk advocacy strategy, preferring to defend the public health safeguards within the system (Hoen et al. 2011). After some discussion, the latter solution gained precedence, and advocacy efforts were directed at promoting the public health safeguards that permitted developing countries from manufacturing or importing generic medicines. The fact that today over 90 per cent of people on antiretroviral therapy in developing countries are receiving generic medicines shows that the advocacy strategy was successful in achieving its goal (Hoen et al. 2011).

Supporting implementation

Arguably, the success of the global campaign for access to antiretroviral drugs over the past decade can, in great part, be attributed to the fact that many of the actors involved – patient groups, health providers, developing country governments – had a practical interest in solving the problem. This meant that short-term solutions, such as drug donations or time-limited discounts, were not accepted because it was clear that in the long term they would not solve the problem. Many of the groups involved in advocacy for affordable medicines were doing so because they were affected, and once generic medicines became available, the same groups began to start providing the medicines to patients. Unless there is a clear commitment to implement the solution, the gains made will likely be quickly reversed. Those opposed (e.g. patent-holders) will promote the failure of implementation as evidence that the solution is flawed, while those in support (e.g. generics companies) will abandon the project due to lack of demand.

C) How students have supported global advocacy to increase access to antiretroviral therapy

The past decade has seen an increasing interest in global health as a discipline, with a proliferation of courses for undergraduates and postgraduates. The importance of advocacy in advancing health benefits is also a growing discipline, with advocacy increasingly being taught as part of formal training for health professionals (Pinto 2008). What is perhaps less well appreciated is the role that students have played as agents of change.

A striking example of the power of student advocacy comes from the early days of challenging antiretroviral patents. Students at Yale University discovered that researchers from the university had discovered a key antiretroviral drug, stavudine. The university handed over the license to the pharmaceutical company Bristol-Myers Squibb, who refused to sell the drug at a fair price to developing countries. Yale students formed a pressure group aimed at shaming the university for their role in contributing to licensing of inventions for profit (Borger and Boseley 2001). As a consequence of this pressure, Bristol-Myers Squibb allowed generic stavudine to be bought and sold within South Africa – and this led to a thirty-fold reduction in the price of the patented drug in South Africa (Chokshi 2006).

This action gave rise to a broad coalition of student activists, such as the Universities Allied for Essential Medicines (UAEM), which is now represented in over sixty universities across North America, with chapters in Europe, Africa and Asia (UAEM 2010). Building on the initial advocacy around stavudine, UAEM's mission evolved to more broadly challenge universities to be more responsive to the needs of developing countries and to undertake research and policy analysis to determine how best to improve access to medicines for poor countries (Chokshi 2006).

D) Conclusions

The scaling-up of antiretroviral therapy in the developing world is one of the most remarkable achievements in global health. In less than a decade, over 8 million people have been initiated on treatment. Novel international funding mechanisms and clear targets for future scale-up have been established, and political commitments are carefully scrutinized by strong civil society activism to hold governments to account (Schwärtlander et al. 2011).

Global health advocacy efforts are often understood as people in well-resourced settings advocating for improved health of populations in disadvantaged settings. The history of HIV treatment activism shows that this is not always the case. Civil society groups in Asia, Latin America and Africa have worked together to support each other's advocacy efforts in an effort to improve access to medicines for all.

This chapter describes a stepwise approach of global health advocacy to increase access to antiretroviral therapy. In reality, progress has not been linear. Access to affordable medicines is again becoming a major challenge as a growing number of people in treatment are developing resistance to first-line antiretrovirals and need to access more expensive, second-line medications (Hoen et al. 2011). The need to focus on HIV care as a global health priority is a concern that requires constant justification. The global HIV programme has been subjected to constant challenges, including pressure from the pharmaceutical industry to limit access to generic medicines, increasing global intellectual property protection that has limited the ability of generics companies to manufacture affordable versions of newer drugs for HIV, competition for global health resources from other diseases, concern that disease-specific funding has been to the detriment of broader goals of health systems strengthening, and changes in political leadership (Mills et al. 2010). Such challenges require constant efforts to gather and publish evidence of the broader benefits of providing HIV treatment at scale.

Global health advocacy focuses on immediate needs and is highly reactive to daily changes in political commitments. In order to develop a broad strategic framework for global health advocacy, it has been suggested that advocates work alongside health policy researchers as a way to encourage more systematic approaches to data collection and policy analysis (Buse 2008). The emerging analytical approaches to health policy analysis will doubtlessly be beneficial to understanding why certain advocacy efforts succeed and others fail (Walt et al. 2008). The challenge will be to connect the lessons learned by academic scholars to health activists, who are intensely focused on responding to the daily, immediate challenges of improving the health and wellbeing of disadvantaged populations across the world.

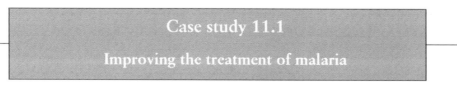

Case study 11.1

Improving the treatment of malaria

Malaria is responsible for around 800,000 deaths each year, mostly children in Africa. In the late 1990s it became apparent that *Plasmodium falciparum*, the malaria parasite responsible for the fatal form of the disease, had developed resistance to the standard treatments, chloroquine and sulfadoxine-pyrimethamine. Countries such as Burundi were confronted with high mortality due to a malaria epidemic in which more than 700,000 cases of malaria and several hundred deaths were recorded in November 2000 (Etchegorry et al. 2001). In response, MSF launched an advocacy campaign to press for policy change (MSF 2003).

Faced with a lack of data and the reluctance of international technical advisors and donors to review treatment strategies, MSF undertook a number of drug resistance surveys to gather data to document the waning efficacy of chloroquine and press for a revision of treatment guidelines. Another treatment, artemisinin-based combination therapy (ACT), had been used in Southeast Asia since the early 1990s, and was highly effective against strains of *P. falciparum* resistant to chloroquine.

The WHO had recommended switching to ACT-based treatment since 2001 (Roll Back Malaria and WHO 2001). Between 1996 and 2004, some forty-three drug efficacy studies were carried out by MSF in eighteen countries to support advocacy for policy change (Guthmann et al. 2008). These surveys all reinforced the need to move away from older drugs in favour of ACTs. However, a number of governments were resistant to making the policy switch, mainly because of the higher cost of ACTs. In order to support African governments to make this switch, international donors became an advocacy target. In 2003, a group of academics from ten countries published an article accusing international donors of "medical malpractice" for continuing to fund older, ineffective treatments (Attaran et al. 2004). Partly in response to these efforts, donors changed their funding policies to support ACT implementation, and ACTs became the first-line treatment option across all malaria-endemic countries.

Case study 11.2
Resurrecting an old drug for African sleeping sickness

Human African trypanosomiasis (or sleeping sickness) is an old disease which was under control in all endemic countries in the 1950s. However, lack of human and financial resources and years of conflict in the most affected countries (such as Sudan, Uganda, Angola and Democratic Republic of Congo) hampered efforts to monitor and control the disease, which re-emerged in the 1980s. Sleeping sickness is a daily threat to more than 60 million people in thirty-six countries of sub-Saharan Africa (Barrett 1999).

Until the late 1990s, the standard treatment for sleeping sickness was melarsoprol, an arsenic-based medicine that caused fatal side-effects in 5 per cent of patients and, due to rising drug resistance, was ineffective in up to 30 per cent of patients. In the late 1990s, an alternative drug, eflornithine, was found to be highly effective against sleeping sickness. However, eflornithine was originally intended as an anti-cancer drug, and when clinical studies for cancer failed, the drug was abandoned in 1999. The WHO, with support from MSF, tried to identify an alternative manufacturer of eflornithine without success – sleeping sickness was a neglected disease affecting poor communities in Africa, and was therefore not deemed attractive by the pharmaceutical companies.

An advocacy opportunity came when another pharmaceutical company launched a drug called Vaniqa, which was an eflornithine-based women's facial hair remover. Ad campaigns in women's magazines stated: "If the mustache that prevents you from getting close is yours (not his), it may be time for a beauty about-face. Millions of women like yourself battle unwanted facial hair." The fact that pharmaceutical companies were willing to manufacture eflornithine as a beauty product, but not as a cure for a fatal disease that killed thousands of people in sub-Saharan Africa, was highlighted in *The New York Times* (McNeil 2001). There is little doubt that the media attention sparked by the Vaniqa launch accelerated eflornithine's subsequent return to production as a treatment for sleeping sickness. In May 2001, the WHO signed a deal ensuring the continued production of eflornithine.

The case of sleeping sickness also led to broader attention to the lack of drug research and development for diseases of the poor. A study supported by MSF found that fewer than 1 per cent of new chemical entities marketed in twenty-five years between 1975 and 1999 were for tropical diseases and tuberculosis (Trouiller et al. 2002). This understanding of the need to address the broader market failure led MSF and partners to establish in 2003 the Drugs for Neglected Diseases Initiative, a collaborative, non-profit drug research and development (R&D) organization that aims to develop new treatments for Neglected Diseases.

References

Altman, L.K. (2006) 'Talking about AIDS, with all the world watching', *The New York Times*, 8 August.

Attaran, A. (2007) 'Adherence to HAART: Africans take medicines more faithfully than North Americans', *PLoS Medicine*, 4(2): e83.

Attaran, A. et al. (2004) 'WHO, the Global Fund, and medical malpractice in malaria treatment', *Lancet*, 363(9404): 237–40.

Barrett, M.P. (1999) 'The fall and rise of sleeping sickness', *Lancet*, 353(9159): 1113–14.

Barry, M. (2003) 'Diseases without borders: globalization's challenge to the American Society of Tropical Medicine and Hygiene: a call for public advocacy and activism', *American Journal of Tropical Medicine and Hygiene*, 69(1): 3–7.

Berridge, V. (2007) 'Public health activism: lessons from history?', *British Medical Journal*, 335(7633): 1310–12.

Borger, J. and Boseley, S. (2001) 'Campus revolt challenges Yale over $40m AIDS drug', *Guardian*, 13 March.

Boseley, S. (2001) 'Drug dealing', *Guardian*, 24 October.

Buse, K. (2008) 'Addressing the theoretical, practical and ethical challenges inherent in prospective healthy policy analysis', *Health Policy and Planning*, 23(5): 351–60.

Chokshi, D.A. (2006) 'Improving access to medicines in poor countries: the role of universities', *PLoS Medicine*, 3(6): e136.

Creese, A. et al. (2002) 'Cost-effectiveness of HIV/AIDS interventions in Africa: a systematic review of the evidence', *Lancet*, 359(9318): 1635–43.

Etchegorry, M.G. et al. (2001) 'Malaria epidemic in Burundi', *Lancet*, 357(9261): 1046–47.

Feldbaum, H. et al. (2006) 'Global health and national security: the need for critical engagement', *Medicine, Conflict, and Survival*, 22(3): 192–98.

Feldbaum, H., Lee, K. and Michaud, J. (2010) 'Global health and foreign policy', *Epidemiologic Reviews*, 32(1): 82–92.

Ford, N. et al. (2007) 'Sustaining access to antiretroviral therapy in the less-developed world: lessons from Brazil and Thailand', *AIDS*, 21(Suppl. 4): S21–29.

Ford, N., Calmy, A. and Mills, E.J. (2011) 'The first decade of antiretroviral therapy in Africa', *Globalization and Health*, 7(3), 1–6.

Forman, L. (2008) '"Rights" and wrongs: what utility for the right to health in reforming trade rules on medicines?', *Health and Human Rights*, 10(2): 37–52.

GlaxoSmithKline (2011) *Global Public Policy Issues: Intellectual Property & Access to Medicines in Developing Countries*. Department of Government Affairs, Public Policy and Patient Advocacy, pp. 1–5.

Guthmann, J.-P. et al. (2008) 'Assessing antimalarial efficacy in a time of change to artemisinin-based combination therapies: the role of Médecins Sans Frontières', *PLoS Medicine*, 5(8): e169.

Hoen, E. et al. (2011) 'Driving a decade of change: HIV/AIDS, patents and access to medicines for all', *Journal of the International AIDS Society*, 14(15): 1–12.

Janssens, P.G., Kivits, M. and Vuylsteke, J. (eds) (1992) *Médecine et hygiène en Afrique centrale de 1885 à nos jours*, Brussels: Fondation Roi Baudoin.

Kasper, T. et al. (2003) 'Demystifying antiretroviral therapy in resource-poor settings', *Essential Drugs Monitor*, 32: 20–1.

Kingdon, J.W. (1984) *Agendas, Alternatives, and Public Policies*. Boston: Little, Brown.

McCoy, D. et al. (2005) 'Expanding access to antiretroviral therapy in sub-Saharan Africa: avoiding the pitfalls and dangers, capitalizing on the opportunities', *American Journal of Public Health*, 95(1): 18–22.

McNeil Jr, D.G. (2001) 'Cosmetic saves a cure for sleeping sickness', *The New York Times*, 9 February.

Mills, E.J. et al. (2006) 'Adherence to antiretroviral therapy in sub-Saharan Africa and North America: a meta-analysis', *Journal of the American Medical Association*, 296(6): 679–90.

— (2010) 'Ensuring sustainable antiretroviral provision during economic crises', *AIDS*, 24(3): 341–3.

MSF (2003) *Act Now to Get Malaria Treatment that Works to Africa*. Geneva: Médecins Sans Frontières, Access to Medicines Campaign.

Perez-Casas, C. et al. (2000) 'Access to fluconazole in less-developed countries', *Lancet*, 356(9247): 2102.

Pinto, A.D. (2008) 'Engaging health professionals in advocacy against gun violence', *Medicine, Conflict, and Survival*, 24(4): 285–95.

Roll Back Malaria and WHO (2001) *Antimalarial Drug Combination Therapy: Report of a WHO Technical Consultation*. Geneva: Roll Back Malaria/World Health Organization.

Schwärtlander, B. et al. (2011) 'Towards an improved investment approach for an effective response to HIV/AIDS', *Lancet*, 377(9782): 2031–41.

Sigerist, H.E. (1941) *Medicine and Human Welfare*. New Haven, CT: Yale University Press.

Tickell, S. (2001) 'Oxfam: Why TRIPS should be scrapped', *Financial Times*, 9 November.

Trouiller, P. et al. (2002). 'Drug development for neglected diseases: a deficient market and a public-health policy failure', *Lancet*, 359(9324): 2188–94.

UAEM (2010) *History*. Universities Allied for Essential Medicines. http://essentialmedicine.org/about-us/history

UNAIDS (2000) 'AIDS epidemic update: December 1999', *AIDS Analysis Africa*, 10(5): 2.

— (2010) *Global Report: UNAIDS Report on the Global AIDS Epidemic*. Geneva: Joint United Nations Programme on HIV/AIDS.

UNICEF, UNAIDS, WHO and MSF (2000) *Selected Drugs Used in the Care of People Living With HIV: Sources and Prices*. Geneva: WHO Essential Drug and Medicine Policy and Médecins Sans Frontières.

Vidal, J. (2001) 'Police guard WHO official after assaults and threats', *Guardian*, 31 August.

Walt, G. et al. (2008) '"Doing" health policy analysis: methodological and conceptual reflections and challenges', *Health Policy and Planning*, 23(5): 308–17.

Wilson, D. et al. (1999) 'Global trade and access to medicines: AIDS treatments in Thailand', *Lancet*, 354(9193): 1893–95.

12 | Teaching global health ethics*

Donald C. Cole, Lori Hanson,
Katherine D. Rouleau, Kevin Pottie and
Neil Arya

Objectives

- To explore pedagogy for teaching global health ethics and its content, primarily to high-income country learners
- To consider the role of high-income country institutions in supporting ethical learning and decision-making in global health
- To stimulate new ideas on assessing the development of ethical global health practice

A) Why discuss the teaching of global health ethics?

Earlier chapters of this book have considered the nature of global health (Chapter 1), key principles that should be considered in the practice of global health (Chapter 2), and challenges faced in global health clinical work (Chapter 7) and research (Chapter 8). We have also examined the journey of learners (Chapter 3) and how global health ethics is incorporated into this journey.

This chapter is written by a group of global health clinical and public health practitioners and researchers who are all educators, actively engaged with learners in thinking about global health ethics in global health practice. We argue that a primary goal of teaching global health is to enhance competency in ethical reasoning. Many students agree (Parikh 2010). Yet a recent systematic review of global health competencies for medical students makes no reference to global health ethics (Battat et al. 2010).

*We wish to acknowledge the contributions of Dan-Bi Cho for searches and feedback; and the Joint Centre for Bioethics seminar participants, particularly Solly Benatar and Barry Pakes for important clarifications.

An orientation towards health for all and health equity is a key characteristic of global health, and hence "learning opportunities in 'global health' should adopt and impart [both] the ethical and practical aspects of achieving 'health for all'" (Bozorgmehr et al. 2011: 3). This is in keeping with the recent call for transformative professional education for equity in health (Frenk et al. 2010), which argues that health professionals need to learn values and leadership skills to act as change agents (see Figure 12.1).

As educators, we have a responsibility to provide practical tools for learners to address ethical dilemmas encountered in a wide variety of activities such as advocacy, public policy, research, education and clinical care. Ethics is a vast subject area, as noted in Chapters 3–5. In the context of already "crowded" curricula in most formal health educational programs, adding the fundaments of theoretical background, ethical principles, normative frameworks such as human rights, and common ethical reasoning processes can be challenging. Nevertheless, learners need to develop a certain depth of understanding of ethical principles if they are to be able to apply more discipline-specific or context-specific ethical reasoning.

In this chapter we focus on how to foster a sustained commitment to realizing principles of global health ethics, with a variety of students across diverse sites of teaching and learning. Throughout, we cite resources and the limited analogous evidence available. We provide examples from our own experiences, some more formally in the form of vignettes. We start with our pedagogical stance, before turning to the contexts and content of global health ethics training. We next consider the roles of institutions in fostering ethical thinking and decision-making in global health (see Chapter 9). We note challenges in the assessment of competency in global health ethics, and some potential future directions.

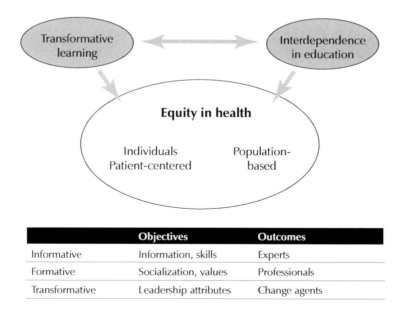

	Objectives	Outcomes
Informative	Information, skills	Experts
Formative	Socialization, values	Professionals
Transformative	Leadership attributes	Change agents

Figure 12.1 Framework for transformative and interdependent professional education for equity in health (Frenk et al. 2010: 53; reproduced with permission)

B) How should we approach the teaching of global health ethics?

Three educational approaches hold particular promise for fostering appropriate attitudes and practices for ethical practice in global health: transformative education, experiential learning and critical pedagogies. These have informed web-based curricula (e.g. Ethics of International Engagement and Service-Learning Project, University of British Columbia), global health certificate programs for undergraduates (e.g. Making the Links, University of Saskatchewan), enhanced skills programs in global health for family medicine graduates (University of Toronto), and approaches in Masters in Community Health Sciences programs (Hanson 2008).

Transformative education can be conceived as moving learners through a spiral of iterative learning (Figure 12.2), such as that laid out by participatory educators in development education (Arnold et al. 1991). This model is aptly coined "education for a change." The teacher assists the learner in making sense of their own experience (1 in the spiral), questioning it (2), discovering new insights (3) and deepening their understanding of how and why things are as they are (4), leading to both key lessons (5) and new actions (6). The teacher/mentor plays the roles of facilitator, advocate and role model. Often the teacher/mentor shares her/his own actions and reflections and encourages expressions of the same by the learner.

Experiential learning can be defined most simply as planned learning from an experience within a clinic, course, program, project or curriculum (1 in the spiral model).

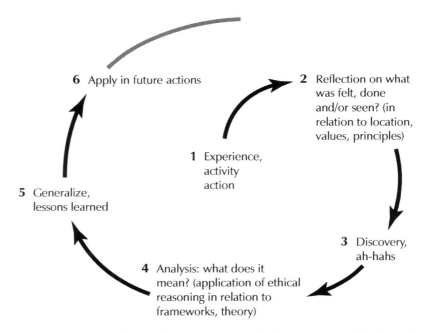

Figure 12.2 A spiral model for fostering ethical practice in global health (adapted from Arnold et al. 1991)

The essential element that moves experience into experiential learning is systematic reflection (2 on the spiral). Service-learning is a type of experiential learning employed in teaching on social determinants of health, health inequities and global health. As described by Deeley (2010), service-learning seeks to provide relevant and authentic professional experiences in real-life settings, with graduated challenges and opportunities for reflection. Service-learning is a pedagogical resource utilized across the globe, and at every level of education (Billig and Furco 2002). A key dimension of service-learning, and one that underpins its ethical foundation, is that the experience and therefore the learning is, in part, determined by the community being served. This element was key in establishing a mandatory six-month practicum in a partner hospital in Malawi for learners enrolled in the enhanced skills program in global health with the Department of Family and Community Medicine at the University of Toronto. In a global health course that was part of the University of Waterloo's distance Master's in Public Health, many students cited the service-learning component as the place they truly learned ethical principles, such as the respect for autonomy and participation. They rated it the best part of their program.

Turning to **critical pedagogies**, Freire's (1970) and Mezirow's (1997) work can assist us in understanding key assumptions, emphases, processes and methods. According to Freire (1970), education can have either an instrumental or an emancipatory purpose. To achieve the latter, educators need to encourage the learner to question, to challenge and to see the exercise of unjust power as problematic (Shor and Freire 1986). The process by which educators can enact Freire's theories is via the "but why" methodology. It seeks an ever-widening and deepening analysis of why things are as they are (4 on the spiral). Mezirow (1997) offers a comprehensive description of the process by which individual learners construe, validate and reformulate their experience through critical reflection, eventually learning to act on their own purposes, values and beliefs, rather than acting uncritically on those of others. Through three major phases of structured or captured learning moments, learners work through (i) a disorienting dilemma, (ii) critical reflection, and (iii) reflective discourse (4 on the spiral). Over time, the associated shifts in perspective lead learners to become more discriminating, to gain a more integrative perspective (5 on the spiral), to think more autonomously, and to be willing to make choices or intentionally act upon these new understandings (6 in the spiral). Case study 12.1 provides an example of such reflection by a resident in a clinical setting.

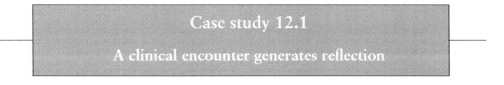

Case study 12.1

A clinical encounter generates reflection

A refugee patient from the Horn of Africa presented at a family physician's office with a relatively new onset of lower abdominal pain. An unexpected positive pregnancy test led to suspicion of an ectopic pregnancy. Sensitive to the discomfort of the patient, alone in Canada with her husband in a third world country, a female resident argued for referral to Emergency, where a gynecologic examination would be performed. The male supervisor insisted on an exam in the office, which the resident performed. The exam did reduce the level of suspicion of an ectopic, allowing an ultrasound to be arranged electively rather than precipitating an immediate Emergency Room consultation. The patient ultimately was found to have a normal pregnancy.

Reflection 1

In a post-consultation discussion, the resident argued that she felt coerced within the teaching hierarchy by her male supervisor, and that the patient could not provide true consent. The teaching physician recognized the gendered, hierarchical nature of his own power over the resident. However, he perceived the calmer office environment, assistance of a translator, and clinical examination performed by a female resident, to be more comfortable for the patient.

Reflection 2

Months later, the resident acknowledged that an emergency referral would have resulted in greater discomfort and would have been less respectful of the patient's autonomy. The teaching physician recognized that his busy office constrained reflection and ethical discussion, producing a less than desirable learning experience for the resident.

C) Where can we engage in global health ethics teaching?

Teaching and learning in global health happen in many formal and informal settings in the course of multiple activities: through discussions in the classroom or at the bedside, during research field work or in conversations using social media and e-learning modules, while undertaking policy development, doing community advocacy, or organizing clinical practice, among others. Because global health as a field is not located "overseas" or in low- and middle-income countries (LMICs), learning global health ethics ultimately can occur everywhere that inequities exist. For example, at the University of Western Ontario, a Marginalized Community Elective involved medical students in refugee clinics facilitating reflection on the contexts and situations from which patients are fleeing, its roots, and the role of high-income country (HIC) governments in fueling or precipitating conflict. As global health educators, our challenge is to seize such learning moments intentionally, set up opportunities for reflection, and support students through the sometimes challenging emotions associated with reflection (Rich and Parker 1995). Learning about ethical engagement works best when it is context- and situation-specific.

Personal experience and social location – the personal learning context – include learners' sense of their social position i.e. gender, race, class, sexual orientation and religion, each of which is often associated with social inequities. Situating such personal contexts is crucial to understanding global health ethics, particularly understanding one's relative privilege in HICs and, as teachers, our own power relative to students. The influence of one's cultural background, personal experience of an LMIC, or powerlessness may afford "insider" knowledge of appropriate ethical practice (see Chapter 3). For example, one of us lectured on global health to Palestinian Master's in Public Health students. After speaking for about half an hour on determinants of health in LMICs, he suddenly realized how the daily reality of his students – checkpoints, roadblocks, frequent tear-gassing as part of the Occupation (Horton 2009) – was outside his usual experience.

Collaboration across different disciplines may provide alternative conceptualizations of health that assist in understanding global health ethics. In the development and health literatures, a broad array of diverse, often opposing views exist on why and how inequities persist. Similar diversity exists on the sources of human values, rights and responsibilities among philosophers and applied ethicists (Benatar and Brock 2011), and among different organizations. The perspective of the headquarters of a humanitarian organization (Schwartz et al. 2010) is different from that of a Ministry of Health or an academic health sciences centre. The impact of cultural and jurisdictional context has been explored extensively for health research ethics (see Cash et al. 2009). Case study 12.2 provides an example where the differences between the perspectives of an HIC research ethics board and LMIC research participants led one of us to modify her teaching accordingly.

Case study 12.2

Cross-cultural perspectives on recruitment into community-based research

A Master's student embarks on a global health research project to document the life histories of traditional birth attendants (TBAs). The project had originated from a long-term relationship between her Canadian supervisor and a Nicaraguan nurse colleague with a thirty-year history of working with TBAs. The Canadian university Research Ethics Board queried how the midwives were to be contacted and recruited – independently by the nurse, with no repercussions for non-participation on the TBAs.

Mid-way through field work, the Canadian supervisor received an exasperated email from the student. The procedures she had laid out in the Research Ethics Board submission had already been violated, ironically by the friendliness and informality that characterized the relationships at the core of the study. The nurse had informally introduced her and her project directly to several midwives, who immediately and enthusiastically embraced her and said – "So, you want to write our story? *Pues, vamos!* (Let's start!)" Every time she had begun to outline the consent procedure verbally, the TBAs became distracted or uncomfortable, with one even leaving the room to go stir the bean pot. Implementation of what was approved by a Canadian Research Ethics Board was considered rude, and quite possibly suspicious or unethical.

Reflection on this experience has led the supervisor-educator to incorporate global health research ethics scenarios that juxtapose formal university ethics procedures with in-field interpretations and she asks students to analyze and pose resolutions to them.

D) When might we teach global health ethics?

The need for training in ethical reasoning and reflection is common across clinical medicine, public health and global health educational programs, hence some joint responsibility should be possible. Timing may be important. At the University of Western Ontario (Marchington and Lappano 2011), ethical issues are raised prior to international experiences during pre-departure training and language courses, as well as afterwards, during post-return reflection and debriefing. At the postgraduate medicine level, a group of Ontario family physicians, including the authors, has developed a curriculum framework for global health in family medicine – emerging principles, competencies and educational approaches – which includes global health ethics (Redwood-Campbell et al. 2011).

For the teacher, part of the challenge is to identify key "teachable moments" in which ethics fundamentals can be applied in the midst of educational activities that may not be focused primarily on the teaching of ethical reasoning. Ethics by definition addresses dilemmas and uncertainty around the right action to take. Global health commonly presents competing values, duties or rights. "Grey zones" are common and are often layered with complex political and cultural issues. One of the key tasks in teaching global health ethics is to enable the learner to become comfortable navigating through decision-making processes in which complexity and uncertainty are unavoidable.

In addition to a solid understanding of fundamental principles, the ability to prioritize principles within particular contexts, and the demonstration of the right level of cultural and political sensitivity and personal reflexivity, are needed. At the other end of the spectrum, learners need to be able to distinguish between flexibility and an overly permissive relativism. The effective teaching of global health ethics should enable the learner to ground decisions in clear, non-arbitrary principles and to apply them deftly in the context of uncertainty. Encouraging learners to disclose their reasoning pathway can help distinguish between relativistic and flexible approaches. Practical guides can be useful, such as a series of questions for students (Pinto and Upshur 2009) which have been incorporated into resident materials for consideration prior to international electives, such as the Public Health and Preventive Medicine policy at McMaster University.

E) Shaping institutions to support the learning of global health ethics

In reflecting on bio-ethics training of medical students, Singer (2003) emphasized the critical place of creating an ethical learning climate or environment, that is, "paying serious attention to role modeling in the learning environment and implementing policies and processes to ensure the learning climate is conducive to ethical development"(Singer 2003: 854). As noted above, cultures and institutions differ geographically, yet share histories of structured inequalities, which pose challenges for ethical global health practice both across and within countries (Benatar and Brock 2011). Academic institutional ethics were a concern of sub-Saharan African doctoral students in a course one of us taught, with both tensions and agreement among HIC and LMIC participants (Case study 12.3).

Case study 12.3

Institutional ethics – perspectives from the South

Funded by a suite of northern private foundations, doctoral students from a variety of universities and research institutes in sub-Saharan Africa came together for an intensive, several-week seminar on conducting population health research in an East African city. Most were lecturers at their own universities, some already actively engaged in research. The session on research ethics around a sub-Saharan African case study of a sexual activity survey went well, but the ethical issues about which students were passionate had more to do with power relations with their supervisors or senior researchers, about fairness amidst hierarchy, and their universities' limited oversight (institutional ethics). They asked:

- Does a senior researcher have the right to put their name as principal investigator on a grant the student mostly wrote? Maybe sometimes, depending upon university policy, said others.
- How about someone in another department who sits on the university ethics committee holding up ethical approval of one's proposal until they get their own research on a related topic done? Most agreed this was unfair.
- Is there some periodicity with which one should be able to meet with one's supervisor? "Regularly" may be defined in some universities, says a

visiting HIC resource person, as including feedback within weeks rather than months.

- Does one's supervisor have the right to put other colleagues' names before yours on a paper you have worked hard on? And as their frustrations continued – How can one obtain recourse around seeming injustices?

No easy answers, but cultural changes in higher educational institutions are needed, agreed all.

Tackling relationships between HIC and LMIC institutions in fostering ethical learning environments is a key part of the Working Group on Ethics Guidelines for Global Health Training (WEIGHT) (Crump et al. 2010), a set of guidelines for institutions, trainees and sponsors of field-based global health training. The WEIGHT group "encourages efforts to develop and implement a means of assessing the potential benefits and harms of global health training programs" (Crump et al. 2010: 1178). Their checklists are a good start for international training partnerships (see Chapter 9). However, promoting "transformation" requires not only programs but also institutional changes (Hanson 2008; Frenk et al. 2010) guided by faculty social accountability–responsibility goals. Good examples of institutional ethics in global health across a range of organizations are provided by Evert et al. (2011), indicating that consciously building ethical approaches to global health is possible.

F) How do we evaluate trainee competency in global health ethics?

The assessment of competency in a domain as complex as global health ethics is challenging, from definition through measurement to interpretation. Yet assessing performance is likely important both for learners and teachers (Singer 2003). We can start with awareness of ethical dilemmas, something pre- and post-session quizzes tap readily. From there, evaluations of pre-departure training (Xu et al. 2011) and course work could assess both the impacts of program offerings in preparing students, and students' understanding of the content. The specific elements might include knowledge of ethical principles, demonstration of ethical reasoning, self-reflection on personal motivations, ability to span levels of responsibility from local to global, and demonstration of cultural competency in decision-making. Some of these overlap with domains that bio-ethics colleagues have some experience assessing (Singer 2003), while others may pose substantial assessment challenges.

How does one assess humility, introspection, solidarity and social justice, as Pinto and Upshur (2009) have argued for in students studying global health? If one connects these broader competencies to those associated with global citizenship, perhaps they could be assessed as externally performed (e.g. when a student participates in acts of solidarity), or as internalized (e.g. via observations of shifting discourse) (Hanson 2008). Overall development in global health ethics might include a summative assessment using a real or fictitious case. Assessment of critical reasoning through vignettes and matched scales has been elaborated for medical ethics by Savulescu et al. (1999). Alternatively, a global assessment by a preceptor could draw upon their own and students' field notes involving critical incident debriefing (Rich and Parker 1995). Self-reflection and key learning moments on global health ethics could be documented, as has been done with passports in other programmes.

G) Future directions in global health ethics teaching

The development of educational tools including web-based resources, scenarios such as our vignettes, and assessment methods should take advantage of the range of learning contexts we have outlined above. For example, the Canadian Collaboration for Immigrant and Refugee Health and the University of Ottawa has launched a Refugees and Global Health e-learning Program to ensure early introduction of global health ethics, advocacy and communication skills for students entering refugee health service learning programs (Pottie et al. 2012). As educational scholars, we should also be evaluating our global health ethics training, including program process, through combinations of questionnaires, focus groups and tutor evaluation rating scales, similar to Goldie et al.'s (2000) assessment of a new medical ethics curriculum. A key step in the teaching of global health ethics will be the involvement of educational partners and preceptors from resource-poor and vulnerable communities, both within and outside the health sciences, to teach and assess learners and our joint programs. As educators committed to mentoring primarily health science learners in global health ethics, we can learn from an experienced philosopher and global health ethics teacher, John Dwyer (2011). Dwyer started reaching the nature of global inequities and theories of justice, but after 15 years he has arrived at emphasizing responsibility and responsiveness, offering opportunities for engagement, and offering hope to learners. May we all do so.

References

Arnold, R. et al. (1991) *Educating for a Change*. Toronto: Between the Lines.
Battat, R. et al. (2010) 'Global health competencies and approaches in medical education: a literature review', *BMC Medical Education*, 10(94).
Benatar, S. and Brock, G. (eds) (2011) *Global Health and Global Health Ethics*. Cambridge and New York: Cambridge University Press.
Billig, S. and Furco, A. (2002) *Service Learning Through a Multidisciplinary Lens*. Charlotte, NC: Information Age Publishing.
Bozorgmehr, K., Saint, V.A. and Tinnemann, P. (2011) 'The "global health" education framework: a conceptual guide for monitoring, evaluation and practice', *Globalization and Health*, 7(8).
Cash, R., Wikler, D., Saxena, A., Capron, A. and Gutnick, R. (eds) (2009) *Casebook on Ethical Issues in International Health Research*. Geneva: World Health Organization.

Crump, J.A., Sugarman, J. and the Working Group on Ethics Guidelines for Global Health Training (WEIGHT) (2010) 'Ethics and best practice guidelines for training experiences in global health', *American Journal of Tropical Medicine and Hygiene*, 83(6): 1178–82.

Deeley, S.J. (2010) 'Service-learning: thinking outside the box', *Active Learning in Higher Education*, 11(1): 43–53.

Dwyer, J. (2011) 'Teaching global health ethics', in: Benatar, S. and Brock G. (eds), *Global Health and Global Health Ethics*. Cambridge and New York: Cambridge University Press.

Evert, J. et al. (2011) 'Global health ethics', in: Illes, J. and Sahakian, B.J. (eds), *The Oxford Handbook of Neuroethics*. Oxford: Oxford University Press.

Freire, P. (1970) *Pedagogy of the Oppressed*. New York: Continuum.

Frenk, J. et al. (2010) 'Health professionals for a new century: transforming education to strengthen health systems in an interdependent world', *Lancet*, 376(9756): 1923–58.

Goldie, J., Schwartz, L. and Morrison, J. (2000) 'A process evaluation of medical ethics education in the first year of a new medical curriculum', *Medical Education*, 34: 468–73.

Hanson, L. (2008) 'Global citizenship, global health, and the internationalization of curriculum: a study of transformative potential', *Journal of Studies in International Education*, 10: 1–19.

Horton, R. (2009). 'The occupied Palestinian territory: peace, justice, and health', *Lancet*, 373(9666): 784–88.

Marchington, E. and Lappano, J.-E. (2011) 'Knight schools spotlight on medicine', Corporate Knights. www.corporateknights.ca/report/8th-annual-knight-schools-results/knight-schools-spotlight-medicine

Mezirow, J. (1997) 'Transformative learning: theory to practice', *New Directions for Adult and Continuing Education*, 74: 5–12.

Parikh, S.M. (2010) 'Global health ethics and professionalism education at medical schools', *Virtual Mentor*, 12: 197–201.

Pinto, A.D. and Upshur, R.E.G. (2009) 'Global health ethics for students', *Developing World Bioethics*, 9: 1–10.

Pottie, K. et al. (2012) 'Refugees and global health: a global health E-Learning program', Canadian Collaboration for Immigrant and Refugee Health (CCIRH) and the University of Ottawa. www.ccirhken.ca/eLearning

Redwood-Campbell, L. et al. (2011) 'Developing a curriculum framework for global health in family medicine: emerging principles, competencies, and educational approaches', *BMC Medical Education*, 11(46).

Rich, A. and Parker, D.L. (1995) 'Reflection and critical incident analysis: ethical and moral implications of their use within nursing and midwifery education', *Journal of Advanced Nursing*, 22: 1050–57.

Savulescu, J. et al. (1999) 'Evaluating ethics competence in medical education', *Journal of Medical Ethics*, 25: 367–74.

Schwartz, L. et al. (2010) 'Ethics in humanitarian aid work: learning from the narratives of humanitarian health workers', *AJOB Primary Research*, 1(3): 45–54.

Shor, I. and Freire, P. (1986) *A Pedagogy for Liberation: Dialogues on Transforming Education*. South Hadley: Bergin & Garvey.

Singer, P.A. (2003) 'Strengthening the role of ethics in medical education', *Canadian Medical Association Journal*, 168(7): 854–55.

Xu, J.J. et al. (2011) 'Assessing the effectiveness of pre-departure training for professional healthcare students working in resource-limited settings', *University of Toronto Medical Journal*, 88: 199–204.

Afterword

Solomon Benatar

Several interlinked global crises in the early twenty-first century are generating serious challenges to the health and wellbeing of billions of people. In order to narrow unacceptably wide disparities in health and diminish threats to our planet and the health of its inhabitants, new forms of societal action are required. Such innovation could transform health care and social systems that promote health into better structured, highly functional, more equitable and sustainable endeavours.

Many of the ideas and much of the content covered in this book, which were discredited or ignored in the past, are now appropriately becoming credible and achieving a high profile. Twenty-first-century thinking is required to solve twenty-first-century problems, just as advances in quantum physics 100 years ago began to reveal answers to questions that Newtonian physics could not provide.

Many of today's young professionals are justifiably critical of the world they have inherited from previous generations, who were swept along by a belief that the world's problems could be solved through a combination of endless economic growth, the pursuit of highly individualistic, consumer-driven needs, and advances in science and technology. The excessive focus on research as the highest goal has also somewhat eclipsed what it means to be a "good" health care professional.

While acknowledging the major contributions made to health and longevity through scientific advances and economic progress, it is arguable that the potential for human advancement globally is undermined by a failure to recognize the crucial need for major changes in the values, discourses and practices that have sustained defective global economic policies and distorted health care systems to the detriment of social justice.

The aspirations of new generations of health professionals, many of whom have a deep commitment to reducing local and global inequities and improving global health, offer the potential for reflexive examination of our goals and visionary collaborative social endeavours. This book provides readers with insights into such new frontiers of ethical and social progress, as well as provocative perspectives on ethical dilemmas in international and global health projects that could foster transformative pathways into a better future.

Index